Gastric Girl

Seven Plus Years Beyond Bariatric Surgery

To Deanna
    All the best +
thanks for your
support + baked
goods!

        :)

        Nichi
            2017

Gastric Girl
Seven Plus Years Beyond Bariatric Surgery

To two extraordinary women:

Dr. Sally Palaian, my therapist who has been so understanding, supportive, patient, and consistent in helping me on my journey. I would not be here without her help. She had helped me realize many truths and goals which allowed me to change for the better. Sally believed in me when I did not believe in myself.

Mrs. Cindy Clemens, who I refer to as "my sister from another mister." Cindy helped me see the woman within and supported me through my evolution. I cannot say enough about her support.

Thank you from the bottom of my heart!

Change does not necessarily assure progress, but progress implacably requires change. Education is essential to change, for education creates both new wants and the ability to satisfy them.

–Henry Steele Commager

Preface

I had a gastric bypass sleeve procedure on October 6, 2009. I was 55 and weighed 438 pounds. This is a description of my experience. The information in these pages started out as notes on my journey with bariatric surgery. The postoperative journey has been a roller coaster ride and by no means easy. I wanted to express the emotional challenges as well as the physical effect that the surgery had on me. In the process, I realized that so many factors and experiences affected my decision and outcome that I had to put the words on paper. I am not a medical professional and my comments are not to be taken as medical fact. Thank you for reading my book.

If you would like to chat with me or send me your story for a possible future book, please contact me at:

willing2becoached@gmail.com

– Nicola "Nicki" Travis

What I Wish I Had Known, Understood, and Accepted

People say to me, "Don't you wish you knew the future? Wouldn't that information make your life easier?" Probably. But then would I learn anything? If my path was already laid out for me to follow, I would not have tried new things or ventured into uncertainty. I might have stayed fat.

As it is, going into my gastric bypass surgery, these are things I wish someone had given me a "heads-up" about.

- My life would still revolve around food (and it does).

- How difficult it would be to eat the required type and amounts of food (still a struggle today—right kinds of food, portion control, and some days intolerance of an item that was previously okay).

- How sights and smells would still be triggers (creating cravings and tummy unrest).

- How angry and jealous I would sometimes get around other eaters (not able to eat the available selections—appetizer, salad, entrée, dessert, and the volume others do). At one point in my life, I could easily polish off a large cheese and pepperoni pizza at one sitting.

- Weight loss would change my relationships (for good and bad).

- My weight loss would make some people uncomfortable (former fat friends who thought I was being judgmental by taking care of myself; it was a negative reflection on them—their perception, not mine).

- Weight loss did not solve my problems (*fill in the blank* _____).

- Being smaller is both exciting and frightening. (Daily life functions are easier but demands on me have changed physically, physiologically, and emotionally. I am now more engaged with people, working out, activities, relationships, and dealing on a deeper levels emotionally—letting myself have those dreams I thought out of reach like a committed relationship.)

- My weight does not define me. (In the past, I felt people saw me as the "fat" girl first, then as a funny, creative, competent individual.)

  I wish I had known -

- How my body would change: sagging skin, remaining fat in some areas, bulges in new places. (Losing weight did not let me contour my body as it traveled this new road. The fat melting off did not result in a hour-glass figure, which eluded me.)

- How to dress to disguise my changing body issues, lumpy body shape, sagging tummy, neck, etc., as opposed to the fat bulging body (trying to judge what styles were flattering and not just a cover-up).

- How to feel comfortable wearing form-fitting clothes reflecting my changing body shape (buying smaller sizes, seeing a new perspective on proportion and how clothes hung on my body).

- How my changing body makes me feel compared to being obese. (Great some days, when I can slide comfortably in a booth at a restaurant, not look around for a "safe" chair, buy clothes in the regular women's shop, etc. Not so great when feeling more pressure to "do things" I have not previously taken on.)

- How overwhelming it is to have so many shopping choices. (I have to learn to try on clothes first, as so many manufactures' sizes vary—going from three or four safe, reliable store choices [Fashion Bug, Avenue, Catherines, and Lane Bryant] to unlimited).

Gastric Girl

Seven Plus Years beyond Bariatric Surgery

Introduction

I am still fat!

I have lost over 175 pounds. By today's health industry standards, I am still obese.

I have managed to keep off 120-130 pounds over the seven years but my BMI and current weight does not equal normal. I continue to struggle.

Why Gastric Surgery?

At a therapy session in April 2009, I was complaining about how little progress I was making with losing weight and how I could not get "started" again. My therapist said to me, "You may have to think about going on disability if you continue down this path."

I freaked out! I had never thought of myself as someone who would have to go on disability due to my weight. I had been overweight or "chubby" since age nine, always on a diet or some kind of weight loss program. I had been in therapy for over 10 years, bitching and moaning about my family, work, and weight. But to actually move to the classification of being "disabled" because of my weight was beyond my comprehension. In truth, I never even thought about the fact that my weight might eventually kill me. These two outcomes—disability or death—never occurred to me.

My aha moment was when my therapist told me that I could go on disability for my weight if I was too depressed to work or socialize. I realized then that the disease of food addiction was winning. I got mad. I could not imagine being defined as disabled—to require assistance, to have a label. I decided that I did not want my weight to define me. That's when I started investigating weight loss surgery. I was able to begin to see that there were other ways of living and to make the choices for a healthier me. After 40 years, I was willing to take a new step.

My Weight History

When I graduated from high school, I stood five feet eight inches, weighed 250 pounds, and had a body mass index of 38. For reference, a healthy BMI for that age and height is between 18 and 24.

I wasn't born fat. I was a "preemie" baby, born six weeks early, weighing just under five pounds. Growing up, my family always said that I never slowed down since my arrival. After my mother was discharged, I stayed at the hospital until I hit five pounds, which was standard medical practice at the time. My therapist has taught me about the issue of "trauma bonds," and the fact that I was not with my mother at this critical bonding time may have impacted my development, both emotionally and in terms of how I related to others.

I grew into a chubby little girl. My older brothers, Paul and Peter, were quite thin. In addition, I wore glasses. I started wearing them when I was two and a half and still do.

I realized I was different. Different from the other members of my family. At first, I thought it was because, with two older brothers, I was the only girl in the house during the early years of my life. The three of us were close in age, all born within four years, which was not uncommon in the 1950s. A third brother, John, came along later, when I was 13.

When I was nine, I remember going to the doctor with my mother, and they talked about my weight while I was sitting in the room. This doctor was not my pediatrician but my mother's doctor. He was thin and stern looking. This doctor scared me. He did not talk to me but frowned a lot and talked in a negative manner. I left not liking this man. My first introduction to the health-care community. I was only nine, but it left a lasting and very sad impression on my psyche.

My mother left the doctor's office with a 1,000-calorie diet for me to follow. None of what transpired was explained to me, but for the first time, I began to realize that my weight was an issue.

From that point on, my food and eating changed. I was singled out at the dining room table about portions and what I could and couldn't eat. I didn't understand what a diet was— I only understood that I was being denied food that the rest of the family could enjoy. The more they restricted my food, the more I rebelled. I started sneaking food from various places in the house: the pantry, the basement storage, and the cookie jar. When food went missing, I was confronted but always denied any role. The standard household joke became "George ate it"—our supposed ghost.

Follow-up visits to the doctor were unpleasant. My weight did not change enough to satisfy my mother or the doctor. Other attempts at weight loss followed. This lasted from ages 9 to 13, until the family focus shifted when my mother became pregnant again, and my third brother, John, was born.

My mother, Katherine, or "Kay" to the family and friends, was always slender. I never saw a fluctuation in her weight. She was five feet six inches tall and maintained a weight of about 125–130 pounds. My mother did not like to eat food. She did not like to cook either. She often remarked she wished she could take a pill to get her daily food requirements. Kay was a daily smoker and coffee drinker. But Kay loved to bake. And we loved it too!

As soon as I was old enough, I started taking over the cooking from my mother. She went to work once John could go to day care. So my job was to start dinner when I got home from school. Kay would select the ingredients for dinner and I learned to put them together for a meal.

Kay tried many ways to control my eating by taking me to Take off Pounds Sensibly (TOPS) and Weight Watchers, working out to Jack LaLanne on television, buying diet aids, and cooking specific foods she thought would help. I think because my brothers were so thin she wanted to solve what she perceived as a potential problem early on.

I felt these activities were sometimes good—because I got to spend time with my mother. Other times, the attention was punitive in nature. I felt "damaged" in some ways because it was so important to her that I change. As time went on, I also felt "not heard."

My mother was not a touchy-feely person. She kept me at arm's length. I got most of what I considered "nurturing" from my dad, Nicholas (Nick). I think that is why I became somewhat of a tomboy.

My parents were both of Yugoslavian descent. My father was born in Macedonia and my mother was first-generation American of Serbian parents. The common country bonds and backgrounds attracted them to each other.

I became quite proficient in outsmarting my mother as far as food was concerned. My chores included setting and clearing the table after meals. That meant I could fake eating correctly at the table and get what I wanted when I cleared the table and stored the leftovers away in the refrigerator.

Our meals were pretty traditional—meat, vegetables, and a salad with desert. Salads were iceberg lettuce, maybe cucumbers, with dressing; potatoes (mashed, baked, boiled) were usually the vegetable. We had lots of casseroles, pot roast, Crock-Pot meals, stews, etc. Very basic meals with little or no embellishment.

My meals were presented without a starch and heavy on salad and protein. I loved mashed potatoes (with butter and gravy) but I could not put more than a large tablespoon of plain potatoes on my plate and feel safe eating in front of my mother. My mother would often cook something just for me as part of the diet plan, and stress to me that she was going out of her way to help me lose weight. One particular meal she made for me was calf's liver—which to this day I detest.

My parents typically retired to the living room to watch the news or read, so the coast was clear for me to feast. I would slice additional portions and eat them as I wrapped up the leftovers. I placed cookies in my pockets for later. I gobbled deserts down while washing the dishes. I ate fast and dealt later with the guilt and anger.

My favorite meals were spaghetti, pot roast, and chicken. The volume of most of our meals was just right for the five of us, with little or no leftovers. Sandwiches with lunch meat, peanut butter and jelly, or Cheese Whiz were my go-to food when nothing else was available.

Looking back at pictures, I was not thin, but I was not obese. I kept asking myself, why should I be treated differently? My brothers were not forced to eat more because they were thin. Their slender body shape followed my mother's side of the family, while I followed my father's side of the family—

more rounded and heavy in the body. Food became a weapon of sorts. First, I knew it irritated my mother that she could not control this part (food intake) of my person. Second, it was about control, mine or hers, over what I ate.

My mother's concern was about image and appearance. The constant scrutiny and lectures from family and friends made food become less about hunger and more about control. I would control what I ate, not anyone else. If she used food as a weapon, I turned food into a game. I ate frozen food from the freezer, found my mother's hidden stash of candy, and when I started getting an allowance, stopped at different stores on the way home from school to buy candy to soothe and feed myself. Plus food was cheap, convenient, and made me feel good for a while.

Now, I was not a slug. I swam and played baseball, volley-ball, basketball, golf, and other sports, but I was never "thin." I was also the chubby friend every group of girls had. I had a very active life, got good grades, worked on the school newspaper and yearbook, went to camp, was in Camp Fire Girls and Girls Scouts, played sports, and went to the YMCA, all very normal activities. But it was not enough for my mother's approval. The weight overshadowed my other accomplishments in my mother's evaluation.

I tried to make my parents happy by doing chores, getting babysitting jobs, mowing the lawn, and helping around the house with my younger brother. Anything to divert the atten-tion away from my weight. Sometimes it worked. Sometimes it didn't.

Shopping with my mother or girlfriends became torture. When I was growing up, the only plus-size store was Lane Bryant, and the clothes were not styled for a teen. There was little selection for school and I would try on outfit after outfit to try to find one my mother would accept. As soon as I could drive, I never went shopping with my mother again. I rarely shopped for clothes with my girlfriends because the stores they frequented did not have my size. I would buy purses or accessories with them but not clothes. I really missed out on the thrill and fun experience of shopping with girlfriends. And this is a pattern that I followed for most of my life.

When my youngest brother was born, I was 13, on the verge of womanhood, and at a time I could have bonded with my mother. Not only was my mother occupied with a newborn, but my two older brothers were on the cusp of college, so the house was pretty chaotic for about two years. In order to make room for the baby, I ended up moving next door to live with my grandparents—my mom's parents—and my room, the castle of a teen girl, became a nursery. I loved my grandparents but I did not want to live with them. They were our next-door neighbors throughout my childhood.

It was not my choice, and I was very unhappy to be shuttled off next door. I moved into the second floor, which had a half bath, a large main room, and a bedroom. Home may have been only a short walk away, but my family felt impossibly far away. I felt very displaced, unloved, and alone. Once again, I turned to food as a friend.

Because my brothers were less than a year and half difference in age, they tended to hang together and ignore me. I still looked up to them but did not interact with them a lot. This was the early 1970s and drugs, rock and roll, and attitudes were definitely laid back. Paul and Peter were at the tail end of the armed services draft process and were more "hippies" than others.

Once both of my brothers, Paul and Peter, were off at college, I moved back home into their room (the upstairs) and resumed living as part of my family. By then I had built up a lot of resentment and anger—the kind of anger a teenager can easily create over perceived unfair family situations. While I loved my family, I thought there could have been a different solution had we talked as a group about it, and I would not have felt displaced and abandoned. Maybe I could have moved to the basement (there was a bathroom) and had a nest there. I would have felt included and part of the family instead of excluded.

And having a toddler in the house with teenagers shifted the attention. We older kids were left to fend for ourselves. We pretty much were on our own as far as getting ready for school, after-school activities, homework, and meals. Paul and Peter were looking forward to going off to college and had already started to disengage. Plus it was the late 1960s and drugs were really becoming prevalent in the community. Many of our neighbors and friends were dabbling in drug usage. I was too scared to experiment.

Growing up I did not always feel I "belonged" in my family. I always had money from jobs and careful planning, so what food I could not get at home, I could buy. I took on the role of second mother to try and stay connected and feel involved with my parents. My mother went to work for the first time since having children (she previously did volunteer work and took care of her parents and family) and my youngest brother, John, started day care. Unfortunately for him, my girlfriends Helene and Patty worked part time at the day care center, and my brother could not get away with anything.

Food stayed my friend through all the difficult times and more in my years of teenage angst (doubts about school, friends, self-worth, future choices on school or careers, etc.). I was a fairly active teenager involved in sports: baseball, golf, swimming, basketball; school activities: newspaper, yearbook, golf league, taking both business and college prep courses; and outside interests: Girl Scouts, camping, photography, babysitting, etc. I was a heavy reader and very social with a variety of friends in the neighborhood and in these other activities.

I had a lot of friends because I liked to surround myself with people. As long as I was busy, I was safe and did not feel shame or a sense of loneliness. I learned early to fill my dance card. So college was busy and frantic at times. I wanted to be a photojournalist since I started taking pictures when I was 10. I earned money doing weddings and portraits both while I was in school and after I graduated. But my parents could not see this as a real job and pushed me into accounting (Mom was a bookkeeper and Dad an accountant) as a safe avenue for a woman. I hated it. After my junior year, I rebelled and switched my major to marketing and made the best of the change. It took an extra year to graduate, but changing majors made my life bearable. When I graduated, I was still living at home—both in order to save money and out of a sense of responsibility for my younger brother, who was then nine.

I graduated from high school, and shortly after, my mother's father died. My parents asked me to move in with my grandmother, again, so she would not be alone. I was in college and the last thing I wanted to do was live with my grandmother, Rose. Out of a sense of daughterly duty (and not being accepted by an out-of-town college), I attended a local university and commuted. I was still helping out with my little brother, John, grandmother, and parents, as well as working part time at school. It was an unwritten rule in our family: daughters took care of everyone.

My oldest brother moved out of state after college with no hesitation, never taking on any responsibility toward the family. The message to the boys was "go out and do what you need to do," while the message to me was to be the "caretaker," responsible and focused on family.

So I moved back in with my grandmother. But this second time, it was more difficult than when I was a kid, living in the relatively privacy and freedom of the second floor. With my grandfather gone, I stayed in the first-floor guest bedroom, across from my grandmother's room. I had less privacy and actual room space to be myself. My grandmother expected me to be visible while I was there. I could not hide in my room, have a majority of my possessions, or display my personality through art work, posters, and personal items. My second stay lasted two years.

I felt at times I was the parent, and I had many arguments with my parents about it. There were no boundaries. I took my youngest brother, John, to his first concert, camping, looking at colleges, etc. I got very mixed messages.

My parents' interest in John focused on his education and physical activity. In third grade, John's Detroit elementary teacher contacted my parents and encouraged them to transfer John to a more challenging environment. He was clearly bored and had capability not being challenged in the Detroit school system.

Since my parents were older (ages 44 and 47), when John was born, they were less down-on-the-floor, rolling-around parents and focused more on providing lots of opportunity-to-learn events. My father retired when John was 15.

I didn't move out of my parents' house until I was 24 because I felt I was protecting my brother from how I was treated. They did not treat him the same as they did me but still were a bit disconnected. My disagreements with my father over parenting roles and arguments with my mother were what drove me out finally. My mother never really championed me one way or another.

Duty and my little brother were my excuses. My grandmother passed away in the late 1970s, and that freed up my parents' attention from her caretaking—but rather than making things better between the three of us, our relationship began to splinter. I was not needed. I got confused as to what my role in the family was. I moved out to my first apartment, which was a one-bedroom, in Detroit, just about six miles from home and a block away from my aunt, who was in many ways a shadow of my future self. She was secretive and overweight.

Through the years, I've tried different weight loss techniques, starting with that medically supervised 1,000-calorie-a-day diet my mom's doctor put me on at nine. I have been on hundreds of diets in the years since: Ayds candies, TOPS (Take Off Pounds Sensibly), Weight Watchers, the grape-fruit diet, the soup diet, the Atkins diet, the all-white diet. When I was a kid, I would exercise to Jack LaLanne with my mother and follow those exercise programs found in magazines.

My most serious weight loss attempt came in 1984, at age 30, when I went to a pilot weight loss program at Wayne State University and was introduced to Optifast, a powder food substitute fasting program. At this time, I weighed 320 pounds. The program replaced meals with protein shakes, and the regimen amounted to less than 500 calories per day. Initially it was difficult to reduced my eating to just five shakes a day. The product was not the best quality and came only in vanilla and chocolate. I had a hard time adjusting to it. We were allowed coffee or tea and sugar-free gum in addition to the shakes.

In the tradition of my eating past, I started modifying the diet plan to my desires. Instead of five shakes, I would substitute hard-boiled eggs and cheese for a shake. I started playing with combinations within the first month. As long as I continued to lose weight no one questioned me about what I was doing.

I was 30 and was very busy with life and work and thought I was on top of my game. If I could just lose weight, I would be *awesome*. I stayed on this program for about three or four months and lost 68 pounds. The huge and sudden weight loss was exhilarating—an artificial high. I was within two pounds of my high school weight. My mind had not caught up with my body's reaction. In the picture below I was about 255 lbs.

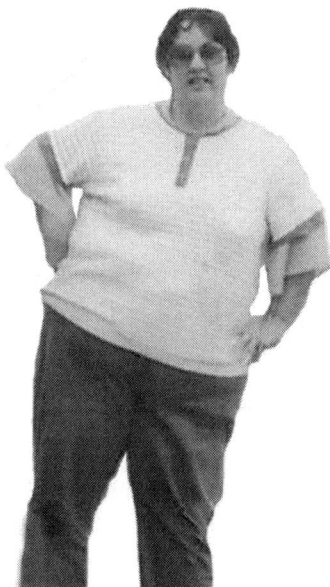

1984

Then I had a job that required me to travel. Being on the road took a toll on my ability to follow the Optifast program. I was always hungry, as my schedule screwed with my timed eating. I felt deprived, hungry, and scared on this program, even more so when I started to travel. I solved the deprivation by adding real food. First I added more eggs to the menu. Next was chicken. I figured these two foods were protein, and how could that hurt? Once I started with solid food, it was too hard to go back to a complete liquid diet. It was too restrictive. I missed chewing.

With solid food, I was less hungry. I felt better. But I was confused by a new set of emotions that followed my success on the Optifast diet. As the weight came off, my body shape changed, I began to receive attention from men—and I was scared. I had been in the "fat friend" category for so long that now that I was in the "datable" realm, I was unprepared.

Part of the Optifast program included weekly meetings to discuss the nutritional and psychological impacts of the diet, and consultations with physicians. The program offered therapy but the group sessions were pretty basic. The meetings did not have the kind of information available now in the health-care community, about the effects of weight loss and emotional ramifications.

Traveling every week for work made it difficult for me to continue in the Optifast program so I dropped out. The weight slowly came back.

Life continued and the scale crept higher. I was working hard and playing hard and ignoring the numbers. Between 1988 and 1992, I lived in Hawaii for a year, changed jobs three times, and finished a master's degree in education (instructional technology). I thought I looked successful on the outside (friends, work, family). From outward appearances, my life had been successful in many ways. I progressed up the corporate ladder, traveled and had many friends.

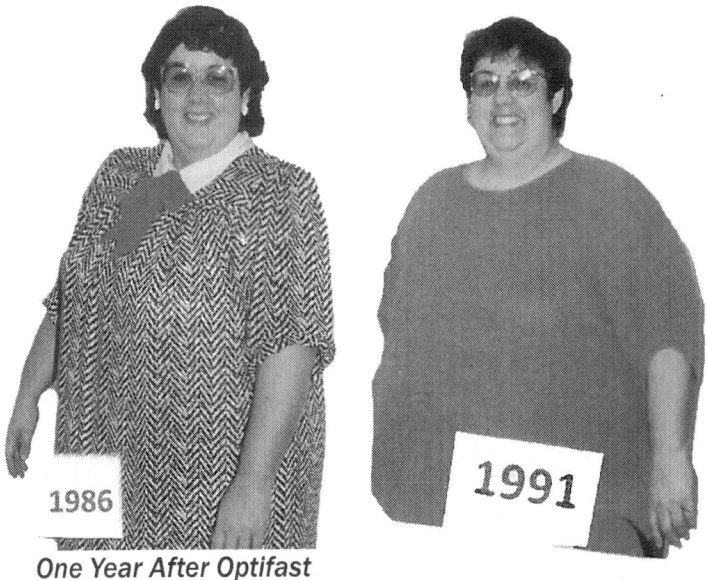

1986

1991

One Year After Optifast

The higher the scale went, the harder I worked and "performed." By "performed" I mean that I hid my frustration, rage, embarrassment, and hopelessness with a fake persona of what a great life I had. I was in sales, professionally, and I was selling the dream to the world and me.

Taking clients out to eat was a big part of my role, and that was where I excelled. If they ate, I could eat comfortably. One holiday season, I attended 33 lunches. Yes, I said 33. One day, we had lunch with one client at 11:30 a.m. and another at 1:00 p.m. Some of the restaurants we used were at the Fairlane Town Center, an upscale venue located in the heart of Dearborn, Michigan (Ford Motor Company territory); the Pool House restaurant (in the pool house of the former home of Henry Ford); Juliano's in the Hyatt hotel; Big Rock in Troy, Michigan; and many others. My theme song was "'Tis the season to be chunky."

In January 2001, at age 46, I reached a new high in my weight: 400 pounds. I was having difficulty breathing and walking. With my therapist's help, I decided to go to a treatment center for help. I went to a facility in Wickenburg, Arizona, for 45 days. This was a multi-addiction rehabilitation center. Food was one of the categories of treatment. Looking back, I wish I had picked a different treatment center, one that focused on food behaviors and not other addictions Of the 60 residents at the facility, only a handful were there to deal with food issues.

But it was at this facility that I was finally introduced to 12-step living for the first time. I came to realize I had huge trust issues, and opening up to someone to help me look at my food issues and feelings felt like getting an amputation. I came to Arizona to get help, but I fought the process. I tried to shape it into something I could control.

In the third week, I allowed myself to consider the possibility of accepting help from someone else and that they might actually know more than I did. It was a tremendous internal conflict within me to deal with giving up control to another person. Trust, hope, and fear, were just some of the feelings I went through in this experience. I allowed myself to hope and opened the door for help a little. I still remained fearful but was willing to try it. It was uncomfortable at times, embarrassing at others. At one point, I had to sit with a counselor at a specific table in the lunch room so my food was monitored. I survived the 45-day journey. I got off caffeine.

I told a few people where I was going. My family knew. I told my boss prior to departure. I did not discuss it with friends and coworkers before I left. I did not have the capacity emotionally to deal with the topic of my weight with people. Once I was there, I did write weekly letters to people at home and work to let them know about my journey and progress. It was also a safe way to open myself up to others about my weight issues.

I returned to work 15 pounds lighter, and I felt healthier and thought I could move forward in the right direction. Part of the recovery requirement after returning home was to attend 90 12-step meetings in 90 days and to continue working with a therapist. I started attending the 12-step program for food disorders, and I continue to do so today. I continued to work with my therapist. While I had altered my course and I was changing myself, my family, friends, clients, and acquaintances did not change. I was fighting the tide, and I struggled to move forward. I did not have enough support in place to even remain at my homecoming weight.

For the next eight years, I struggled with my weight, 12-step program, therapy, and life. I quit a very lucrative sales job because I felt it was contributing to my poor choices. I have been jumping from small ventures and different jobs since

2004. Some were successful, some not. As I was building my support internally and externally, I was still eating to deal with life.

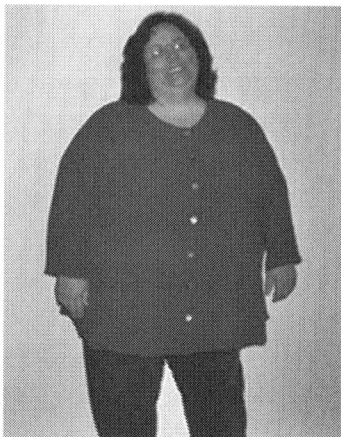

Work, 2004

Weight inching higher.

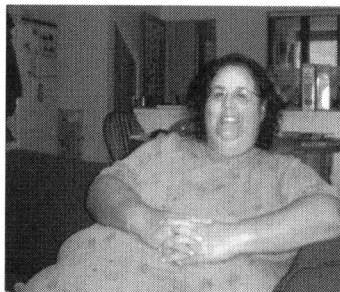

October 2007

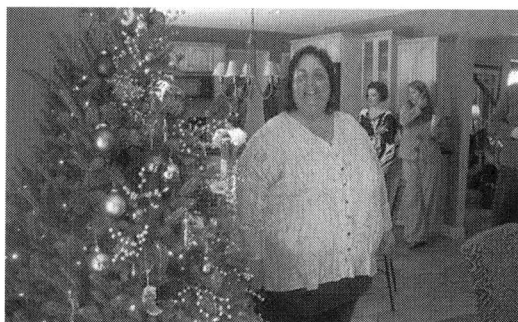

December 2008

Decision to Have Gastric Bypass Surgery

In 2009, I hit a new all-time high of 438 pounds. My BMI was 66. I could no longer ignore what I was doing to myself or expect to have any kind of quality of life.

I decided to have gastric bypass surgery in June 2009. I thought with all my therapy, workshops, and other treatment, I should try what I had been avoiding. I imagined that this time I would be *forced* into changing my eating habits, that it would be the "cure" I had hoped for— and one that would last forever. I thought that I could not circumvent the surgical affects by cheating and binging.

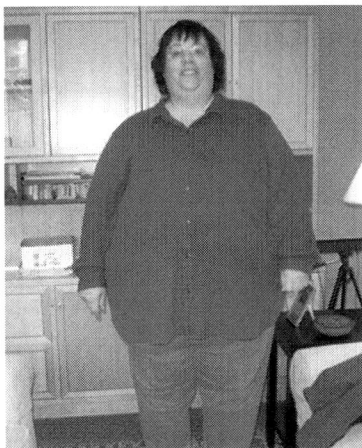

I hoped that my decisions about food and eating would become a routine, normal matter. I thought I would not be able to harm myself anymore. And for a while, all my hopes came within my reach.

The Process

Did you know that over 250,000 people have bariatric surgery each year? I have known of this surgery being offered in the United States for over 15 years. In the United States that equates to 3,750,000 people having surgery for weight. The United States population is approximately 320 million people. This means 1 in every 853 people have this surgery.

Pre-Surgery Orientation

My bariatric program took place at the Warren campus of the Henry Ford Macomb Hospital in Warren, Michigan. I attended a bariatric orientation session in June 2009 to obtain information and learn about surgery options, issues, and concerns. They gave me a three-inch binder of information to review and digest. After the orientation session, I made an appointment to meet with the hospital bariatric nurse coordinator and see what the next steps were. I choose this program for two reasons: it was named a "Center of Excellence" by the American Society for Metabolic and Bariatric Surgery (www.asmbs.org), and the all-inclusive price covered the surgery, anesthesiologist, hospital stay, and nursing care.

The bariatric nurse coordinator took my vital physical information, medical history, and photo during an intake meeting. We reviewed my next steps from the orientation packet, which included (1) choice of surgeon (I got to choose—I could pick someone I could relate to), (2) type of surgery, (3) getting a physical, (4) taking a sleep apnea study, (5) having a psychological evaluation, and finally (6) meeting with the surgeon. I was asked if I had any questions; I didn't at the time.

Fulfilling the steps was not hard. I made the necessary appointments and started the ball rolling.

Physical Examination

My physical exam was pretty basic, much like a school physical. A nurse recorded my medical history, blood work, and height and noted my weight. My blood pressure, temperature, allergies, and medication information were taken. It took about 45 minutes and I was out the door. I guess I expected more.

Sleep Apnea Study

I scheduled my sleep apnea study for a Monday night. What a crazy experience! I had been a restless sleeper for a while, and having all the wires attached to my head and chest made me anxious and even more restless. The study monitors your heart rate, breathing, and level of sleep and correlates them. I learned during the process that lack of adequate sleep could lead to weight gain. The study revealed that I had some dramatic issues with my heart and breathing sequencing. They were so serious I had to return on Tuesday to be rechecked. I returned for a second night of testing.

On Wednesday, the clinic called and ordered me to get a breathing machine immediately. The urgency of the staff member alarmed me. I got upset at the lack of information and explanation about why I needed it so quickly. I was not given the results of the test, only told to get the breathing machine ASAP.

I called the nurse coordinator and explained how the staff at the Sleep Clinic had scared me with their urgency, directions, and information. She understood my fears and reassured me that she would contact the clinic and get back to me with more information about moving forward. I felt much better after that telephone call. The nurse coordinator called the clinic and set up an appointment for me with the doctor in charge of the sleep apnea studies to get more clarification. I went to the appointment and learned how frequently I stopped breathing at night and that those gaps in breathing also caused the heart to stop beating—a very serious combination. The doctor explained what was occurring inside my body, how a breathing apparatus would solve the disruption problem, and how my weight was the contributing factor. But If I lost weight—at least 50 pounds, he said—I might not need the machine forever. Hearing that my heart was stopping regularly during the night was frightening. How had I not known this previously? Would my primary physician have known this? I walked out of there much more informed and relieved at the potential solution.

When I got the breathing machine, a continuous positive airway pressure (CPAP) device, the clinic staff person made sure it fit properly and walked me through the usage process. It felt like a scuba diving mask, confining and weighing heavily on my face. I didn't like that feeling.

What a learning experience. The first machine was temporary and did not use water. The clinic provided another machine, which was to be my permanent machine. It had a water component on the newer model. I liked the original model better. The second machine was noisy. The water reserve ran out during the course of the night. I would wake up with a dry mouth and have to add more water to the CPAP. I learned to keep a bottle of water at my bedside. Sometimes I just took the damn thing off and tried to sleep without it.

The more I talked to other people about using a CPAP, the more I found friends who had been using CPAPs for years to help with their breathing and sleeping.

Once I got used to it in the first two weeks, I seemed to sleep better. It had never occurred to me that my weight was a major link to my sleeping difficulties and insomnia over the last several years. I stopped using the machine after two to three months when I had lost roughly 60 pounds (January 2010). I was sleeping deeper and waking up more rested.

Psychological Evaluation

My psychiatric evaluation would determine if I would be approved for surgery in 2009. It consisted of interviewing with a psychologist and completing an online psychological test that took about 40 minutes. We discussed the history of my life as it pertained to my weight. I listed the various methods I had used in the past to lose weight (Optifast, 1,000-calorie-a-day diets, Weight Watchers, Atkins, etc.). Included efforts on my part was hiring a personal chef, seeing a nutritionist, and diet pill supplements.

I also discussed the gastric bypass procedure (previously the lap-band) with the psychologist. I had read about it 10 years earlier when it was fairly new in the United States and was a much more invasive procedure. In 2000, I had gone with a girlfriend, Diane, to Port Huron, Michigan, where the lap-band was first offered in Michigan. We attended the orientation session offered by the hospital to determine if it was an option for us. There were close to 200 people there. The Port Huron hospital staff talked about the procedure, recovery time, insurance costs, the steps to take, and how to sign up. They also presented three different patients who had the surgery and were in various stages of recovery (four weeks to six months). It seemed like a miracle cure at the time.

My friend decided to pursue the surgery as a result of the session. I was much more skeptical, plus I was about 80 pounds lighter than my 2009 weight. Diane signed up and went through all the steps and was scheduled for a lap-band surgery in November. Sadly, two days prior to surgery, she did not have insurance approval. Unwilling to pay for it herself, she backed out. Insurance approval was much more difficult to get then. Diane subsequently got the insurance approval but never went back for the surgery.

Over the last 10 years, gastric bypass surgery has improved tremendously. There are three main surgical procedure choices and all can be done laproscopically now, allowing for tiny incisions through the stomach rather than major abdominal surgery: gastric bypass, lap-band, and gastric sleeve. The hospital stay is much shorter, the risks are reduced, and the surgery is easier.

Surgical Evaluation

Once all the pre-surgical requirements were met, my case went before the Henry Ford surgical board. They evaluated me as a potential patient and the feasibility of my success. Once the bariatric team decides that you are a viable candidate, a surgical date is assigned. Then an appointment is made with the selected surgeon to discuss the actual surgery. Not everyone gets approved. Some patients are rejected because they do not demonstrate a willingness to follow the pre-surgical diet, the changes in food behaviors, or changes in attitude. Others do not qualify because their health changes and risks factors are too high.

Surgical Consultation

I met with my chosen doctor, Dr. Carl Pesta, in August 2009. We discussed the procedure, what to expect during surgery, the hospital stay, and aftercare. He set a goal for my weight loss based on my height and general health and explained what support I should expect from him and the team (his office, the hospital and the bariatric center staff) and reminded me to reach out for any reason, with any question or health concern. I had a ton of questions on the recovery process, reintroducing food into my system, and timeline for weight loss. Dr. Pesta addressed all of these questions.

Dr. Pesta was kind and reassuring about the surgery, my fears, and expectations before and after surgery and answered all my questions. I had met this doctor at an orientation session and spoke with other surgical patients, who praised him and his office staff and felt confident with his skills. He was the youngest of the three available surgeons. I was not worried about the surgical aspect of the process.

My goal was to get below my high school weight of 250 pounds. I had not seen that number ever but came close at 252 in 1984. Dr. Pesta said that my weight loss depended on how well I followed the program after surgery and the additional steps like change of food choices and exercise required. The surprising information I got was how they measured success. If you kept off 50 percent of the targeted weight loss goal long term (five years or more), you were considered a success.

Additional pre-surgical criteria must be met during the prep phase. The initial process is to follow a strict food plan as provided by Henry Ford Hospital two weeks prior to surgery to clean out and shrink your stomach. Weight loss is expected to occur. If there is no weight loss, the surgery can be cancelled at the surgeon's discretion. I lost 15 pounds prior to surgery. I followed the diet to a T because I wanted the surgery.

Decision Time—Type of Surgery

I chose to have the gastric sleeve type of surgery. The "sleeve" procedure means two-thirds of your stomach is removed. The stomach ends up looking like a banana.

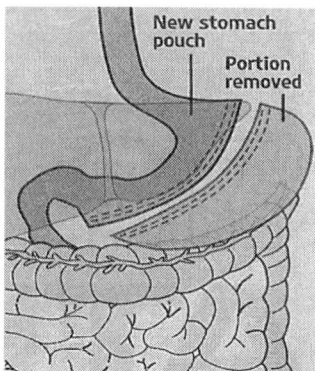

Of the three available procedures, this one is not reversible. While this procedure had been around for two years, Henry Ford doctors had not offered it prior to 2009. After doing some research of my own, I opted for this choice. I looked at the pros and cons of each surgery, the success factors, and the recovery process. In addition, by using the remaining one-third of my stomach functions, it allowed my body to process nutrients, vitamins, and minerals, which the other two options could not provide, as the stomach was totally bypassed. It offered the least side effects, had less aftercare requirements, and had the same hospital stay: one to two days.

On October 6, 2009, I was one of three patients to have the gastric sleeve surgery performed at Henry Ford Macomb Hospital Warren campus for the first time.

Home Preparations before Surgery

Not only did I have to prepare myself, I had to prepare my home for my new adventure. I emptied out all my regular unsafe foods and junk food and replaced them with protein shakes, Jell-O, broths, soups, and items that would get me through the first two post-op weeks. I wanted to binge badly and eat everything in sight, but I followed the presurgery diet preparations carefully. I was too afraid to be rejected for surgery.

I wondered how long I could stay on this path. I wondered what I would really be able to eat. I was scared. I prepared by making lists—lists of what I hoped would happen, of my fears and goals for clothing fantasies, physical activities I wanted to be able to do, and more.

Finally, I completed my most important pre-op task: I took my official "before" picture, at age 55, and weight of 438 pounds.

Family and Friends

I minimized my announcement before the big day. I really did not want to tell anyone. I was afraid I would back out. The only people I told were my younger brother, John, and two girlfriends, Angela and Karen. I was acting the non-emotional, don't-need-your-help gal. Plus, I had trouble discussing my weight with family members. It had been a "hands-off" topic for a long time.

I did not want to discuss my decision with family and get feedback that would upset me emotionally or cause me to doubt my choices. It was the first time that I felt in control of my body, weight, and future. My mother would drill me with questions and dissect the process, location, doctor, and related choices. The remaining family members did not discuss my weight or body issues because I never let them. My friends understood my challenges and emotions about food much better.

I finally told my family members two weeks prior to surgery that I was having the gastric bypass, after John's insistence. He wanted to make sure my family knew of the surgery and the drastic turn my life was about to take. My mother, Kay, was quite worried and scared for me, but hopeful. For many years, she badgered me about my weight and then gave up on me. She was glad to see me take action even if she was unsure of the outcome, but she was concerned about my ability to look after her as her primary family aide.

I figured a short stint in the hospital would not alert anyone. I was not working and it would not be noticeable to casual acquaintances if I did not see people for a few days.

I think that I would not have told any of my family without my brother's insistence. I did not want to talk to them about the decision and get into any "deep" discussions about why I was having the surgery. We were not a family who shared feelings. When I did tell the family, few questions were broached, and the main concerns were about the safety of the surgery.

Surgery

During the steps prior to surgery, I thought I was processing all the information, but looking back, it was a bubble, a bubble of denial of my physical condition floating just out of my sight. The bubble was the mind space I was in going forward. I was disconnected, going through the motions, and taking in the information but not really owning it: the surgery was going to define my relationship with food and what I ate for the rest of my life.

As a child and as an adult, I had created many scenarios and games around my insane eating habits. (For instance, it did not count if no one saw me. As long as I ate the healthy meals I could have a treat after. If others were eating the food I wanted, I should be able to have a piece. Once I started binging, it did not matter, etc.). This surgery would take away much of that fantasy world. I had used food to reward myself, numb myself, as a weapon or control (I can eat this whole pizza, cake, box of cookies, etc., and no one can stop me), and as every other form of emotional escape.

I got to the hospital on time with my girlfriend, Angela T. I was required to bring my CPAP and get weighed prior to surgery. I was moved into a room to be prepped for surgery, and I felt pretty calm. I had been in hospitals in the past for minor surgeries and had no horror stories. So the surgical part did not scare me.

The hospital had a separate section for bariatric surgeries, a floor with about seven rooms. The furniture and accommodations were for larger people. I felt at ease and that the staff understood the difficulties and frustrations an overweight person faced in everyday life and medical situations. The staff was incredibly compassionate.

When I arrived at the hospital, I had to weigh in. If I had not followed the two-week pre-surgical diet and lost additional weight, the doctor could cancel my surgery. I was also instructed to bring my CPAP machine. Luckily, I lost 15 pounds in the last two weeks. I was good to go. In prep-op, the surgical nurse set up the IV and other medications. By this time, my mother and another friend, Karen, had arrived in time to see me off to surgery. Then I was out for the count. I remember leaving the staging area and no part of the actual procedure. I woke up in my hospital room a few hours later. No memories of anything, thanks to good drugs!

After surgery, I felt very little pain—I was just thirsty. I was able to get ice chips and eventually popsicles. I was pretty loopy too from the drugs. I had some issues with my breathing, as I had a hard time clearing out the anesthesia. The staff was concerned with my oxygen readings and kept me on oxygen the whole two days I was an inpatient. To avoid blood clots, compression stockings, which squeeze the legs gently every 30 seconds were put on both my legs.

I did not feel different. My pain from the six one-inch incisions was minimal. In fact, there was no irritation or swelling from the incisions. By the end of the first day, I walked down the hallway of the hospital floor. I had not experienced the true eating/surgery changes or challenges yet. The recovery aspect was similar to any other surgical experience.

The following inpatient day included checking of vitals, especially my breathing levels, more walking, checking of the incisions sites (five one-inch incisions and one slightly longer one where the camera was used), and bathroom action. In order for me to go home, all of my bodily functions had to work properly. At the close of the second day, a physical therapist came by to ask me to climb a short series of steps. If patients can accomplish that task, they're cleared for release. I did it! The next day I went home.

I honestly had very little pain or discomfort. The incisions and the shots I had to take for 10 days did not faze me. The process of drinking the protein shakes and other liquids was the challenge. I managed the first two weeks on protein shakes, Jell-O, and clear liquids. Graduating to soft foods took a while. I was scared of being sick and throwing up or "dumping."

My mother, who was 84 at the time, came to the hospital with two of my girlfriends during the surgery. Mom was thrilled I came through the surgery well. I was relieved that she was okay with it and seemed to "get" what I was doing for future health. We were dancing around talking about my weight. Due to the short stay, I did not have any other visitors. After I had the gastric bypass sleeve surgery, I allowed myself to talk about it with people in my circle. As time went on, I got more comfortable discussing the surgery and my general weight and health issues. I went from wary silence to blathering. I had made a major life-changing choice, and I think I wanted external reassurance that I did not invite when on previous dieting choices.

The reality of this decision to have the surgery did not really sink in until a good two months later, when I was able to resume a fairly regular eating regime. In the first stages after surgery, I did not want to eat. It was hard to get the correct amount of protein in every day. Initial food of liquids, protein shakes, and broth gradually progressed to soft foods: blended soups, pudding, and oatmeal. We were encouraged to add foods at a pace that we could handle. Protein first. Vegetables and fruit followed. Avoid carbs and sugary items.

Some unpleasant and unexpected outcomes:

- Nothing tasted the same to me.

- Surgery removed my enjoyment of foods I once loved.

- And to be honest, I am rarely hungry now.

Post-surgery / Life at Home

I hoped that life would be simple once I got home, but there were lots of rules, steps, and requirements to follow. First and foremost, I needed to take medications to prevent any health complications post-surgery:

1. I had to give myself twice-daily injections to prevent blood clots for 10 days.

2. I had to consume 60 grams of protein daily.

3. I had to drink 64 ounces of liquids a day.

4. I had to walk.

5. I could not drive until the follow-up visit with surgeon.

6. I had to answer a lot of questions from everyone.

I managed the first weeks at home fairly well except for a few dietary mishaps as the days went on but nothing major. I was considered a model patient.

Weekly Support Group—At the Hospital

People in the support group represented patients from just out of surgery to those who were two to three years post surgery. The great majority were women, and the average patient was about two to three months post surgery. I found out that some gastric bypass patients never attended these sessions. Even with the surgery, some people are ashamed to admit that they could not lose weight on their own and kept their surgery a secret from family, friends, and coworkers.

I learned from this group how to get the required food in, whether it was at the liquid stage, soft foods, or regular food. Even though we were provided with a two-inch binder with much of this information, it was more helpful to hear people who had gone through the process speak about it and what they did. Tips on how to get the maximum protein, recipes, food choices and brands, protein bars, which bariatric supplier was better, where items might go on sale, comments on certain brands, and good websites were all offered up during these sessions. Some patients shared food samples so others could determine if it was worth the price given how the texture and taste was to their palette.

But the group changed and became less helpful as time went on. While I realized that after their initial adaptation to the eating process, people would not need any further advice, I was sad to see them gone. The support meeting was geared to the first three months out of surgery and not long-term recovery. I wanted more than ways to consume the required food amounts, different food choices/selections, and recipes. I was fairly well past the post-surgery pains and early digestive problems and was now feeling different. I stopped going.

Though there are many blogs and corporate websites available to access and get information about surgical recovery, I preferred the person-to-person sharing experience. I think there should be a similar ongoing program like a 12-step program for bariatric surgical patients. While there is a 12-step program that addresses food compulsion, it does not include the challenges that a bariatric patient encounters. I have also experienced some bias in the 12-step program for having taken what is deemed a "shortcut" by having gastric surgery.

I think that having the surgery was a life-saver for me. Attending the 12-step program for over eight years had not helped me turn my food addiction around to a healthy place. The 12-step program offered understanding and support that I desperately needed but not "recovery." I still attend meetings regularly to maintain a healthy mind and receive support during my continued journey.

First Holiday Season after Surgery

As Christmas 2009 approached, I worried about the holidays and visiting people. How was I going to eat at the festivities? I certainly did not want to eat real food, as I was scared about what worked and did not. Not much food agreed with me yet, since I had just graduated to solid food and was still eating soft foods like pudding, cottage cheese, and soups. I was sure I would try a few cookies and find out how bad it might be. The Food Addict mind was still lurking.

But first I went off to Florida for 10 days. I was already 60 pounds lighter and felt pretty good overall. This venture was to Jensen Beach, Florida, to stay at my sister-in-law's family condo with my friend Angela T.

Food was a quandary. I tested different items to see what worked, what stayed down, and what I could tolerate. I had just weaned myself off the protein shakes and liquids, but food—food food, solid

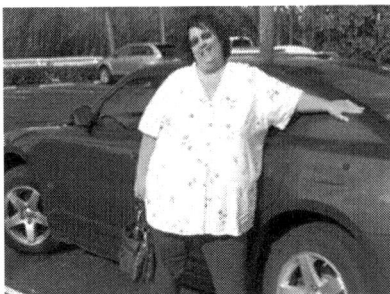

December 2009

food—scared me. I was not feeling hungry and yet I had to feed my body to burn off the pounds and maintain my health.

Travel was easier than it had been before the surgery, and there were some nice moments: I did not need the seat belt extender on the plane—a new success! Once settled into the condo, Angela T. and I went off to the grocery store to stock the fridge. Grocery shopping was tricky. I did not want to buy too much because I had not figured out the portion size I could handle, but I did want to have choices. I was not really thrilled about eating. I really preferred not to eat at all!

It was a good trip. We had no definite plans except to relax, use the pool, and walk on the beach. That worked out fine. Angela was pretty athletic; she liked to work out more than I did, and she could walk long distances. I could not. But I could swim. And the weather was good for 6 of the 10 days, so I used the pool. The complex had a workout facility, which Angela T. used while I swam. I attempted to do my water aerobics routine but I was still not that flexible after surgery.

In my journal, I wrote: "I noticed that I am cold all the time after surgery. I used to be called the furnace because I was always warm to the touch regardless of the weather. I would usually go without socks year round. But now, I am cold all the time and my bones hurt." I am sure it has to do with the amount of food I was eating—or rather not eating. I started a collection of sweaters and hoodies, a first for me. Even in Florida, I was wearing layers. Sensitivity to cold was not covered in the bariatric surgery orientation manual.

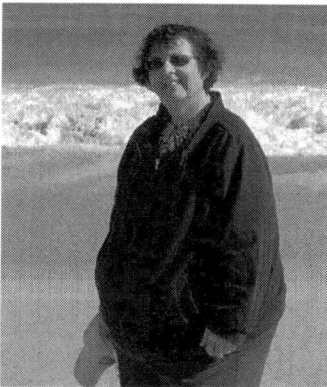

December 2009

I learned the achiness in my bones might be due to the chemical changes in my body and decreased calcium levels. I have not been too successful with taking my supplements. Eating has been enough of a challenge, and adding those vitamins and calcium to my daily routine is worse. Wearing extra layers and complaining about my aches and pains while in sunny Florida made me feel so old!

I still wasn't hungry, but I forced myself to eat. I carried peanuts with me so I always had something to eat, and I lived on frozen lemonade as well.

Overall, the trip to Florida was a great beginning for the new me. I felt so positive about the future, and I was sure that this path was the ticket to health. But I was also scared. I was afraid I would sabotage myself, eat the wrong food or not enough food, or just plain screw up. Oddly, I was more obsessed with food than ever before. Hmmmm, how did that happen?

A Few Surprises

As I progressed through the months after surgery, I had some surprises. My first was having a menstrual period three months after surgery—and three years after going through menopause. Imagine my panic—it had been over three years since I had had a menstrual period and the last thing I wanted to worry about was a potential or future pregnancy. (The surgery was sometimes used to help women who were overweight be able to get pregnant, as weight was determined to be a deterrent to conception.) I immediately called the nurse coordinator and told her my story. I was reassured that this was not uncommon. In fact, the orientation book stated that the surgery could sometimes increase fertility in women. Whew! That was a close call. Luckily, that occurrence was a onetime deal.

My second surprise after reintroducing foods in my diet was my total intolerance of bacon or pork. I loved bacon and pork chops and pork roasts, but now they did not love me! The meat was just too dense, and if I tried to eat it, I suffered from "frothing" indigestion, where the food does not stay down and leads to vomiting. Not pretty.

Nausea and Vomiting

Nausea and vomiting are the unpleasant results of not following nutritional guidelines. I would have many stomach difficulties if I did not plan around the following:

1. Taking enough time whenever eating and/or drinking.

2. Drinking fluids with a meal; drinking too soon before or after a meal?

3. Eating too much.

4. Sufficiently chewing solid foods until they resemble a puréed consistency.

5. Lying down too soon after a meal.

6. Eating foods that are hard to digest, such as dense produce, dry meat or fresh bread.

7. Progressing to the next stage of the food plan before being cleared by the surgeon to do so.

Frothing

After having the gastric sleeve procedure, you retain a third of your stomach—in essence, a pouch. As the new pouch heals, mucous is sometimes built up. In some people, the mucous backs up into the esophagus and causes frothy clear vomiting. Generally, this is short lived and resolved by the third month or so after surgery—but not for me. I found foods that were dense in consistency also caused this problem. In addition to pork and bacon, I also had to give up steak—and I love steak!

Dumping (Diarrhea)

"Dumping" syndrome occurs when a large load of simple carbohydrates such as those found in table sugar, ice cream, milk shakes, and sugary desserts enter the small intestine too quickly. Since my anatomy has been altered, foods high in simple carbohydrates enter too quickly, which in turn causes the "dumping" symptoms (a quick dash to the bathroom). Consuming foods high in fat and drinking water with meals can also cause similar symptoms.

Lifestyle Changes

Changing my lifestyle meant changing my behaviors and that is one of the most difficult challenges for me. Changing daily food habits is one of the most important factors for my long-term health. And let's face it: if your body mass index is high enough for you to qualify for bariatric surgery, you have developed deeply distorted behaviors around food. You can change or stop many bad habits, but you can't do without food. I still have to eat. My challenge is to change *how* I eat.

My previous eating behavior was to starve all day, surviving on soda pop until late afternoon or early evening and pigging out on dinner (all the courses—appetizers, salad or soup, entrée, and dessert). Other times, I would eat cereal, popcorn, or crackers as a dinner substitute. Occasionally it was a medium or large pizza. Lots of carbs, sugar, and sodium went into this body. Now I had to reprioritize and make it protein first (at least 60-80 grams daily), then vegetables and possibly fruit.

I heard the same logic from doctors and nutritionists for years. But putting those changes into practice is wholly another matter. Alcohol, gambling, and drugs are addictions that you can actually avoid 100 percent—and being sober requires doing so. Food? Not so.

Personal Accountability

Being responsible for my eating habits, choices, and actions remains an ongoing challenge for me. I find I am more involved with food and the eating process than ever before. I used to ignore all the rules about healthy eating and just did whatever I felt at the moment. Now I have to plan. That is the biggest challenge to me: PLANNING! In my 12-step program there is a saying: "If you don't have a plan of eating, you plan to fail." I have to plan what I am going to buy and how much to cook and make the right meal portions to prepare a variety of dishes. Without variety, I get lazy and look for the easiest thing to eat. In my case, it is a premade snack (Armour Snackables) which contains 10 grams of protein in the cooked ham variety (ham, crackers, cheese, and a mini Nestlé Crunch bar) or Oscar Mayer Lunchables, which have 14 grams of protein. This is my emergency meal when I am too lazy to prep food or cook a meal. Plus it is very portable. (Yeah, like that is the most important feature, to tote food around all the time—ha.)

Being honest about food is *hard*. It means looking inward and acknowledging what food was to me, what it did to me, and how I have abused both food and my body. Lying about food since age nine gave me about 40 years of practice. Lately, I try to get real about food and portions. Habits are hard to change. But they change one day at a time. Record keeping is highly suggested. Not only do you track what you eat and if it is (1) enough, (2) timely, and (3) a healthy choice, I have to acknowledge what I am really eating. Honesty. Making it real. My behavior and lifestyle determines my success. As my nurse coordinator says, "If you bite it, write it down".

Being real means:

1. Hitting ideal weight is unlikely even with surgery. If you lose 50 percent of your goal, the surgery is working.

2. Seventy percent of our calories should be protein.

3. Soda pop is the worst thing—it can stretch your stomach.

4. Carbs trigger hunger.

5. We (surgical patients) need a minimum of 60 grams of protein but should aim for 100 grams of protein daily.

6. We (surgical patients) need to focus on how we feel—the feeling of fullness, so we can recognize it. Hunger vs. "appetite" (whether you feel hunger).

Grazing is high risk, eating with no plan or purpose, resulting in higher calorie intake. Learn to ask yourself:

1. What time of day do I graze?

2. What am I grazing on and how did it get there? (In the house, office, drive-thru, car, etc.)

3. What activities are encouraging me to graze?

4. What type of food am I craving (salty, sweet, chewy)?

5. How do I feel when I want to graze?

Identify your triggers. You cannot rely on *willpower* alone.

1. What are your 5 trigger foods?

2. What is going on emotionally?

   H = hungry

   A = angry

   L = lonely

   T = tired

These emotional first letters spell HALT.— which is what you should do. This is a term describing feelings used by my 12-step program. Food temptation will always be there; it is just a question of whether I go there again and sabotage my progress. The road to success involves making important changes in behaviors. By having bariatric surgery, I decided to travel a new route from the one I had previously traveled. To proceed on the new route, I know I must make new kinds of choices each and every day.

Some choices:

1. Eat meals at regular times each day.

2. Ban eating directly out of serving bowls or pans!

3. Resist tasting when preparing food.

4. Leave food on the counter or stove rather than serving from bowls on the table.

5. Eat in the dining room or at the kitchen table, not in front of the television or in the bedroom.

6. Serve food on a small plate or in a small bowl.

7. Chew each bite 20 to 30 times to a puréed consistency.

8. Stop eating at feelings of fullness.

9. Prepare a shopping list and stick to it!

10. Shop for groceries after you eat.

11. Read the labels and look for foods low in calories and fat.

12. Avoid high-calorie snacks and beverages.

13. Use environmental control to make your environment friendly to your weight loss goals.

14. Avoid snacking.

15. Plan physical activity in your daily life.

16. Record keeping will help you know if you are on track.

17. Monitor your fluid intake.

18. Use solid protein and high-fiber fruits or vegetables to help fill your stomach pouch.

19. Avoid eating triggers. Do other things to avoid your triggers.

Record Keeping

Daily food records are important to manage your weight. Each day you should record what you eat, your vitamins, fluids, and how much physical activity you have. Record keeping eliminates the mystery behind why you lost or gained each week. The records give you instant feedback on how you are doing. My records help me see if I am getting adequate nutrition and hydration. The categories to track are

Water intake	Exercise
Caffeine intake	Fruits and vegetables
Carbonated beverage intake	Protein shakes
Vitamins	

Even though bariatric surgery decreases the amount of food I can eat, I still have to make good choices. *The temptations will still be there*. Best defense: a good offense! I have to look carefully at my environment at home and at work and where I go and what I do for fun and relaxation. I need to eliminate the things from my environment that lead to an unhealthy path. Identify the foods that trigger me to overeat, throw them out and definitely don't bring them into my environment. Create my environment with things that will support a healthy lifestyle; buy a treadmill; good walking shoes; always have the proteins, fruits and vegetables on hand.

Problem Solving Early

If there are problems in accomplishing my plan, I can't

throw up my hands and give up. If plan A doesn't work, make plan B. For example:

1. If you normally exercise after work, but you know that you'll be doing some overtime, you will probably need to get up an hour earlier to get your exercise accomplished.

2. If you know that you are going to a potluck dinner in the evening, you will need to bring food to the potluck that you know you can eat (in other words, don't rely on others to provide the food you know you must have).

So I know that to be truly successful, I have to be vigilant about:

Exercise

Changing My Lifestyle

Keeping Daily Records

Solving Problems

Hospitalization after a Fall

In 2010, I fell as I was walking into the Troy Community Center to do my water aerobics on an icy February morning. To avoid smashing my face into the glass doors, I twisted away from the door as I fell to the ground. I herniated a disk and fractured a vertebra as a result—not something I would recommend to anyone. The only positive aspect was that I weighed 90 pounds less than before my surgery, and was not as embarrassed to be picked up by the EMT attendants on a backboard.

But the 12-day hospital stay that followed was a real blow to my weight loss progress. The incident set up a whole new set of problems with my food, which I never anticipated.

I was taken to an excellent hospital, Troy Beaumont, which provided wonderful care for my back injuries—but the staff was clueless when it came to dealing with a fairly new post surgery bariatric patient (a little over four months). I was lucky I did not need a nasogastric (NG) tube. Bariatric patients cannot have NG tubes for breathing, as there is no place for the tube to go. (The NG tube goes down the throat to the stomach.) It is recommended that postsurgical patients wear a warning bracelet or necklace tag stating the health alert.

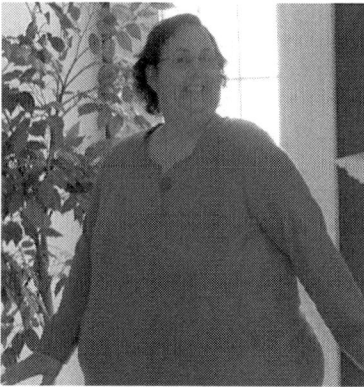

February 2010

Every heavy person's fear is the embarrassment of not fitting in a "normal" situation or environment. Being transported by ambulance is stressful. Not fitting in the ambulance would be overwhelming.

I encountered many problems at the hospital. First I was required to lie flat on my back, which affected my ability to digest food, resulting in acid reflux big time! In addition to the pain and anti-inflammatory medications, I was taking medication for stomach relief. I needed to maintain proper calcium and potassium levels because eating was difficult.

Now understand, taking pills can be difficult for a bariatric patient depending on the size and the quantity. I regularly took four pills a day for other health reasons and to accommodate the additional pills required was a struggle. I had to convince the nurse that I had to space out the drugs if they wanted them to be successful. Pill taking remained a challenge for the entire 12 days I was there.

Food and beverages were delivered at the same time. Food portions were too large and the wrong type of food. All beverages were provided with straws.

A bariatric patient cannot eat and drink at the same time. Eating and drinking have to be spaced appropriately for safe and comfortable consumption. Straws cause air bubbles in bariatric patients' stomachs and are not recommended.

Food choices were limited. Even after I met with the nurse

and dietitian, I could not get the correct food selection and portion size and settled for protein, juices, and crackers with an occasional Popsicle.

The hospital offered these standard dietary meal choices:

1. Clear liquid diet

2. Full liquid diet

3. Transitional diet (bland, easily digested food)

4. Mechanical diet (swallowing or chewing problems)

5. Low residue diet (high fiber)

6. Consistent carbohydrate diet

7. Neutropenic diet (low blood count or medication interactions)

8. Cardiac diet (low fat, low cholesterol, no salt)

9. Low sodium diet

10. Low fat diet

11. Renal diet

Not one fit me. A secondary issue was the frequency of eating *necessary* for a bariatric patient (six times a day) was difficult for the hospital staff to understand and administer.

At one point, a CAT scan was ordered and I was to drink a 12-ounce Caltrate beverage for the test. A bariatric patient can only drink two to four ounces at any one time. I was advised to drink as much as I could before going for the test. I wondered out loud to the staff if the consumption amount would affect the final test results. No one had an answer.

Dealing with the pain of the fall was actually easier than the discomfort of eating and getting my nutritional needs met during my hospitalization. After I was stabilized, I was transferred to a nursing home for rehabilitation, as it was deemed I could not go home and function well alone. I lived alone, and the bedrooms were on the second floor. Basically, I was miserable both stomach- and back-wise. I received an epidermal injection that eased the back pain enough so I could make progress. I could get out of bed and start walking again.

Nursing Home Care (Post–Hospital Stay)

I was transferred to the nursing home for a two-week stay in March and was happy for the assistance and physical therapy I received. It really made a difference to receive the care after my fall. With the staff's help, I was progressing from a wheelchair to a walker and then a cane.

I was thrilled when they weighed me, because I lost about 25 pounds in the hospital over the 12-day stay—which was much too fast a rate—as a result of the uneven eating. The nursing home staff helped me maneuver, dress, go to physical therapy, and learn to walk again. My balance was affected by the fall and the continued weight loss.

Meals

I meet with a dietitian three times during my two-week stay, and we never resolved the food issues, which carried over from the hospital. While I stressed that protein was important and gave a few suggestions, my meals ended up being scrambled eggs, tuna salad, and grilled cheese with orange juice, cottage cheese, and Jell-O daily. I managed to get saltines as well. The smell of the food and the medication put me off eating. It was a struggle to just take my medication.

There were usually three meals a day, at 8:00 a.m., noon, and 6:00 p.m., with a lot of water and ice available throughout the day. Shakes such as Ensure or Boost were available, but those are for increasing calorie intake and protein, so they are high in sugar and aimed at elderly patients to maintain their weight. The menu did not offer a lot of sugar-free items.

I was pretty miserable at this time, but in the back of my slightly demented mind was my food addiction. It lurked and suggested that eating less than nothing was a sure way to lose the weight faster. I survived mostly on orange juice and the saltines. I would ask people to bring me food so I could have some variety. Sometimes I could handle it, but other items got rejected after a bite or sip.

The following is an example of the Nursing home's daily meal selection.

Breakfast	Orange juice, hot/cold cereal, sausage patties/links, pancakes, baked apples, oatmeal
Lunch	Vegetable soup, barbecue pork on a bun, potato salad, butterscotch pudding with topping (alternative: hot turkey sandwich, mashed potatoes)
Dinner	Chicken and dumplings, spinach, wheat roll, strawberries, and bananas (alternative: Salisbury steak, mixed vegetables, banana, potato)

My post-op food program emphasized protein, protein, and protein—then vegetables and fruit. These menu items had a lot of sugar, salt, and fat. Since many of the residents were elderly and needed to maintain their weight, it was good for them but not the best for a foodie and recent bariatric patient like myself. Otherwise, the stay was uneventful. I received great treatment and physical therapy and was able to go home with a high level of confidence. After leaving the nursing home, I did get physical therapy visits at home for another few weeks, which helped tremendously.

But I left with the feeling that the health-care community needs to be more knowledgeable about the challenges of bariatric patients.

After about a two-and-a-half-month break caused by my injury, I went back to the hospital-based support group and wanted to reconnect with those who had been so helpful and those who had surgery around the same time as myself. I wanted to compare notes and see how successful people were with food management and weight loss. To my surprise, there was only 1 person left that I

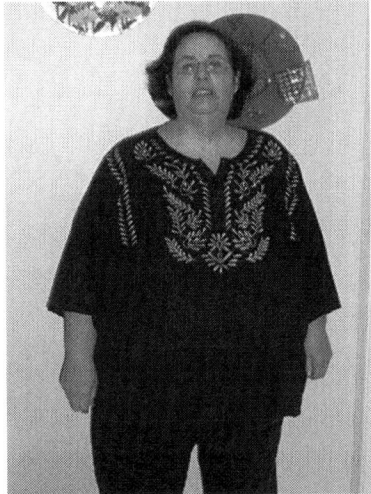

April 2010

recognized in the room of 19. Most of those that I had met in earlier sessions no longer attended.

While I realized that after initial adaptation to the eating process, people would not think they needed any further support, I was sad to see them gone.

Anger

I was about eight months out of my surgery and I found I got angry at my inability to eat volumes of food. I missed taking a big bite out of a hamburger and eating all the courses of a meal and then having desert. Previously, it was easy for me to finish off a 12-ounce steak, a salad, a potato of some kind, and maybe another side dish with a chocolaty desert. I hated seeing other people eating food, enjoying it, setting it aside when they were sated. It brought up so much resentment—first because they could eat what they wanted and second I now saw and felt how my detachment and food behaviors got me to this point in my life.

Now I have to choose which food I will eat for my meal, or have a small bite of each item—and that's all. No longer can I polish off a bag of chips with dip. No more can I eat half or more of a large pizza. No way can I devour half a carrot cake at my leisure. It just sucks!

Then I remember I was 145 pounds less than when I began this journey. I can still savor those items in smaller portions if I choose. But my bad food habits, or "stinking thinking," do not go away quickly. I had to take an in-depth look at the emotional and psychological issues that contributed to my weight gain in the first place. I was not going delude myself into thinking that just because a person loses weight their personal issues will dissolve too. The emotional baggage doesn't shrink with the rest of your body. Dealing with the baggage in my head has been much more difficult than healing from the gastric bypass surgery itself. I have to come to terms with the fact that much of what I feel was formed when I was a child. Twenty years of therapy and self-help did not erase the ingrained thought patterns.

I blamed myself for lack of control and for reacting to others who judged me. Being fat is considered a sign of weakness or laziness. People say, "Just push the plate away or just eat half of what you order." Other sayings that irked me were "You have such a pretty face . . . If you would just lose some weight you would be so much better," and "Just stop eating and you will lose weight." (Really? I didn't know that. How rude!) And fat is the last arena of discrimination. I have always worked jobs where weight was not a big deal—just my performance results. So as long as I produced revenue, I was golden. My last few jobs were different. I worked for slender or normal-size people, and I could feel their discomfort radiate when I sat near them or we had to travel together. I felt like I encroached on their space and wanted to squeeze into a ball and be smaller. I would get angry yet feel I had to make them feel better, to make them feel safe, rather than take care of myself.

I think that the hardest group of people to deal with is medical professionals. They are educated in the ways of treating weight gain and loss from a clinical perspective—not the psychological and emotional issues that often underlie the physical condition. Over 40 years, I have been given and tried hundreds of "diets" by doctors and other health-care providers. And guess what? Diets don't work. And yet the medical profession continues the same course of treatment. It suggests that something about the whole process is screwy.

Food choices, environment, stress levels, and relationships all affect how I process my feelings, and that relates to my food consumption. Happy, I eat; sad, I eat. I just eat. Therapy has helped me understand the thought process behind my choices about what I eat, how much, when, and how frequently. And with understanding, I hope to dissect or disrupt those paths that lead to unhealthy behavior and to change them.

Those old paths of eating and acting out when I could not handle my feelings were destructive. I now recognize those paths when I stray, and I can recover and turn away from them more quickly. Otherwise I will hold onto my anger and distrust and continue to abuse food rather than use it for nutrition and health.

I carried the anger inside me like a black hole. I used to imagine myself in a warehouse-like room with tall shelving to the ceiling, and everything black. No windows, no light, and no way out. And I was stuck. I was stuck because I was unwilling to ask for help. If I asked for help with my food issues then it meant that I had a "problem" and had to deal with it and with "outsiders." As long as I denied myself help, I could ignore the problem. But weight is visible. It really is.

So I learned to cope. And one way was to disassociate from the problem. I stepped out of my body and pretended to be at a weight that was acceptable in my mind. It did not matter that I was 70 pounds overweight in reality. Then 120 pounds. And then 170 pounds, and finally 238 pounds overweight. Now how could I ignore that?

The mind is a powerful tool. The more I stretched it, the more it adjusted just like my body. As long as I could move and do daily normal activities, I blocked thoughts of my weight. It was not until I was short of breath walking around that I started to be present in my body. Now I had a constant reminder of how bad off physically I was becoming and own it.

In the past, I would check out. If I was entertaining a client or meeting someone for the first time, I would go on the offensive and be charming and engaging, making the meeting all about them. I would do things to get them to see past the physical size of me and see the funny, charming, and insightful person I thought I was at the time. So much of the sales work I did included wining and dining the customer. During that one holiday season when I attended 33 lunches for business, not once did I think about scheduling meetings around a conference table instead of a restaurant booth or finding a healthier alternative. I used work as an excuse to justify my excessive eating.

During those meals, I would encourage the client to try anything, including desert—and if they indulged, then I convinced myself that I could eat what I wanted. I even had one client with whom I established an "eat dessert first" ritual. It started during the holidays when the client saw the dessert tray and said, "I need to save room for that," and the waitress said they were almost out. So we decided to have the dessert before they ran out. Thus began a ritual that persisted for two years. Crazy, crazy, crazy! But when you have a food addiction, inventing weird ways to get food is the norm.

And what did I desire? Well, the biggest thing I wanted was connection—connection to people. Working in the service industry is like being part of a family. I was always offering services, and in my mind that brought me closer to people and gave me a sense of intimacy. I grew up the only girl in the family, and I felt I had to take care of everyone—whether that was true or not. I played the mediator, the protector, the victim, the thief, and many other roles in order to feel connected.

We had a large chest freezer in the basement and I would raid it to get treats that were denied to me. Cookies and candy that were stored in the cupboard went missing. With three kids in the house, it became "George" who was the mysterious thief. The funniest thing was that while I was restricted at mealtime, it was my job to clear the table, do the dishes and put the food away. I would bide my time and eat off the plates before washing them. As I put food away, I would take the leftover portions and stuff them down. If it was a cake, I would cut a slender piece and gobble it down.

If my mom made chocolate chip cookie dough (usually a double batch) I would eat the raw cookie dough in little dribbles, sometimes eating as much as a quarter of the dough. Cookies baked and in the freezer were high on my favorites list. (And our family's chest freezer is still working 43 years later.)

So I learned early on not to admit to *what* I ate, much less *how much* I ate. So I stopped paying attention to volume. Any spare money I had I spent on treats at the corner store on the way home from school. I took great care to discard the wrappings before I got home.

Drive-through are the world's worst invention. Not only are they quick, but the drive-through is fairly anonymous. And there are so many choices that you can drive through several in a day. I would drive through and buy whatever I wanted. The window clerk would not care if I were buying for myself or a family of 10. Coupons were another way of justifying my purchases—because how could I *not* take advantage of a good deal? Two for the price on one was a favorite of mine. And of course I ate both rather than setting one aside for the next day. The food was warm, cheap, and available. Yum!

Now, I am not blaming the businesses out there that cater to food service, but there are too many choices and most are unhealthy. A person has to take responsibility for their choices. I know I didn't. And that is how I got to this place.

Today, when I am out and about and I see a really obese person, I so want to go up to them and tell them my story. But then I think, would I have been responsive to someone doing that to me? No way! Thinking about and seeing obese people keeps me in check. I don't want to slide back into the fog.

There is an emotional letdown as the weight loss becomes a normal occurrence and the newness begins to wear off. It's easy to experience depression after gastric bypass surgery. The very-low-calorie menu or maybe my body's way of slowing down after major surgery can cause this. So to monitor this, I kept seeing my therapist, who has been a constant support over the years. (I originally went to therapy to lose weight. Boy, was I clueless about the journey ahead.)

Depression

I used to think I was depressed all the time when I was at my heaviest. It was a good reason to keep eating. And it made sense to me. I started to see a difference in what I called depression and it was actually an attitude of indifference. Not caring about myself or the foods I ate increased my disassociation. I stopped caring about the type of food, the volume, and the effect. I stopped seeing myself.

The topic of depression came up in the pre-op orientation and in the support group. We were advised to be realistic in our expectations and in our actions. The doctors and the nurse coordinator said, "Don't jump into fantasyland by thinking all your problems will disappear if you are thinner." While my quality of life would improve thanks to the surgery alone, as the patient, I still had to take an active role in my recovery. In my notes, I wrote: "Food is everywhere and sometimes I feel like the kid pressing on the glass looking in at all the baked goods. I am kind of mourning the loss of food. I have a lot of fond memories and have certainly eaten my fair share of food."

I first went to Dr. Sally Palaian in 1988 with just one goal—lose 100 pounds. I paid cash for my sessions, as I did not want anyone to know I was going for help. I found Dr. Palaian through a flyer about a women's health group. Dr. Palaian was kind and willing to help me. She tried to tell me it was not just an issue of losing weight but the rationale behind how I arrived there. It was not what I wanted to hear.

Therapy did not last long (two to three months). I took the "change jobs" approach, thinking that would solve my problems. It did not. I started a new position in health care in October 1988. I lasted at this job 15 months. The position was not what I expected so I made a contingency plan of going back to graduate school. I started graduate school at Wayne State University in January of 1990. I had worked in the field of technical training for a while and decided to get the credentials to move up the ladder. The program I picked was a masters of instructional design (education). This could be considered another "avoidance" technique for dealing with my food issues.

Graduate school classes were in the evening and it was impossible to take more than two at a time. So I had my days free and time on my hands. I got a call from a former colleague and was subsequently offered a job with his company. I was working full time and going to school. Much too busy to deal with eating issues.

In summer 1991, I got a call from a former coworker about a contract job opportunity in Hawaii. I had to laugh. Could this be real? It was. The work was on Oahu for the Hawaii Medical Service Association (HMSA), creating training for their new claims system. The initial assignment was a year. I was offered the position. It was a crazy time. I had my thesis due and was almost done with school. I figured out a way to submit my thesis and complete the last class of my education program and go to Hawaii. I left for this work in July 1991.

While I was in Hawaii, my allergies ramped up and I was having constant respiratory problems. The doctor I saw put me on inhalers and allergy shots. I survived. My contract ended in Hawaii and I was eager to come home. I was offered another year contract but only wanted a six-month one. Since we (HMSA and I) could not agree, I left Hawaii and came back to Michigan.

For whatever reason, I did not stop using the medication for my respiratory problems once I got home. After a few months, I started having bouts of insomnia. I found myself unable to make simple decisions about work assignments, outings, and daily chores. After three days of no sleep, I drove myself to the local hospital emergency room and was treated for an "asthma" attack with a nebulizer treatment and recommended to see a doctor.

I knew there was more going on that just lack of sleep and contacted Dr. Palaian and arranged to see her. I had my mother drive me because I felt unsteady and unsure of my reactions. This was late fall of 1992. Dr. Palaian recommend that I see a psychiatrist to evaluate my medications. That was a primary step in treatment—to make sure of no ill medication interactions. Next, she and I talked about what was going on and I agreed to start therapy again.

I went to the psychiatrist as soon as I could get in. She determined that the medications I was taking typically created a high anxiety level in people and even panic attacks. She thought the "asthma" attack I had was really a panic attack and that the treatment utilized would help either condition.

I no longer needed any of the allergy medication now that I was back in Michigan. It was removed and I received a medication to relieve the anxiety and depression that I was exhibiting. Within a weekend, I felt so much better. I knew that I was finally taking care of myself. I was asking for help.

After that initial visit, I started therapy with Dr. Palaian.

The fact that I continued my therapy after surgery has helped enormously. I get to use my therapist, Dr. Palaian, as a sounding board for new stresses and experiences. She helps me normalize those moments. And she reminds me to continue to remember how far I have come and to have gratitude for all the work I have done, something I easily forget. Another path I can take now is one of awareness. Through therapy with Dr. Palaian for over 20 years, I can identify how I will react in certain situations ahead of time and make plans to keep me safe and not crash and burn emotionally. Dr. Palaian has been a great lifeline through my initial baby steps of therapy, self-realization, and getting out of denial and into real recovery.

Clothes

I have this new body and all my old clothes hang on me. I was hesitant to start buying things because my body was still changing but I needed help. There were clothes that I had never worn with tags, and I had since skipped past that size.

Clothes were everywhere, the bed, dresser, on the door jam, the floor. I had never let anyone in on my clothing purchases and never sought anyone's opinion. I hired Joi Sherman, a clothing consultant, in August 2010 to help me dress. I did not have a clear view of myself anymore.

This was a process suggested by my therapist. Joi had me try on every single piece of clothing, including shoes and purses. And in the end, I could only keep about a sixth of all the items. The rest either went to friends or the Salvation Army or was sold on eBay or Craigslist. It was a unique experience for me to let someone in to "see me" and to see my real body shape, to see how my clothes fit this changed body of mine. For most of my life, I shopped by myself or ordered things online rather than sharing the experience or be embarrassed by trying on clothes with someone looking.

A prerequisite for this clothing session was that I purchase new bras so that my clothes would fit properly and hang correctly. Good undergarments are crucial for good fit. So I went and treated myself with a visit to Harp's in Birmingham, Michigan, a well-known lingerie shop, and purchased three new bras. And I was quite surprised at what size I actually was (but I am not telling).

My closet was full of clothes with price tags still on them, clothes I had bought with the hope I could wear them someday. I had held onto some for years. The sad part was that by the time I went looking, I had lost enough weight that I had actually passed by some of the sizes without an opportunity to wear the items.

I was devastated to let go of a particular business suit. It was unique in color and design and cost $500. I never wore it. Once we had determined what items could to stay in my closet, I got a lesson in styling the items I had and how layering works. A week or two later, we scheduled a shopping trip so I could fill in some clothing gaps. We met at Kohl's, where my consultant, Joi, had done some pre-shopping and had about 20 items set aside for me. Finally, I could shop at Kohl's for clothes—not just purses and house goods, but all types of clothes.

I ended up with five new pieces: a shell, two blouses, a sweater, and a pair of pants. All pieces were in colors of black, white, and gray or a combination thereof as a foundation for the future. Something Joi recommended to have as the basics. A bit somber for me in terms of color choice: I preferred reds, plums, and blues but these were good, basic pieces.

Later, I ventured off to Parisian, a nearby department store, on a mission of my own. I needed a black purse. And I was open to buying other items as well. I have gone to these stores and purchased non-clothing items—purses, jewelry, cosmetics, gifts, etc.—all my adult life, but never really looked at the clothes or the different lines carried in this store. So to the women's department I went. Instead of the limited options from Fashion Bug, Catherines, Avenue, and Lane Bryant, I had options like Evan Picone, Calvin Klein, Ann Taylor, and more. Totally new and exciting! But it was also a weird experience, and I was a bit overwhelmed by all of the choices available. I managed to buy one blouse and two purses—a little victory. I followed the consultant's rules about color and style. And I used coupons.

In my journal, I wrote: "I have 3 closets in my bedroom and currently only have clothes hanging in the smallest one. My choices have greatly expanded as I have shrunk. It was now December 2010 and I still used just the one closet. Being on a small budget and not wanting to buy too many clothes as I continued this journey, I got quite excited to find a pair of shorts for $4.99 and Capris for $9.99 for a Florida vacation in December."

Luckily, the 12-step program's convention in Detroit in October 2010 offered a clothing exchange. People donated clothes and you could go in and take anything you wanted, and as much as you wanted. I picked up a few items for down the road. Earlier in the year, at a similar clothing exchange held at the hospital, I picked up a winter jacket and coat that has been well used.

In this new life after gastric bypass, it seems you need to buy new clothes every month. One good tip is to buy at Goodwill, Value World, or Salvation Army, and donate the clothes back when you are through with them. I really want to shop but must remind myself to hold off, as I still plan to lose more weight.

I did find some other stores similar to Salvation Army that allowed me to fill in gaps as I lowered my clothes size. I was really happy when a new plus size resale shop opened in April

2011, only a few miles from my house. Items I was unable to sell on Craigslist or eBay went to their new home, and with the store credit, I scored some new threads.

December 2010

I had lost 175 pounds by December 2010. I was within 13 pounds of my high school weight. It was unnerving to say the least. I was afraid. I was afraid I would sabotage myself. I was so close to my goal that I had a hard time comprehending it. My overall eating was still limited, but with meals consisting of more protein and increased frequency, I was better off than six months earlier when I struggled to eat two or more meals. My food choices had expanded, and I felt more comfortable eating out. I was feeling good and enjoying my new clothes.

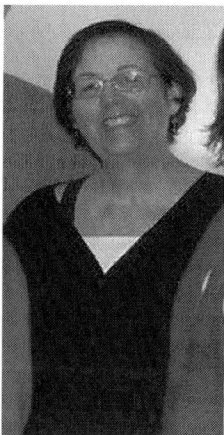

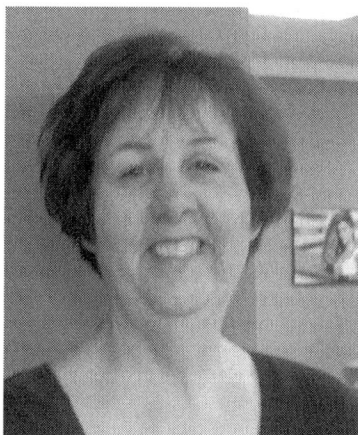

December 2010

I was still unemployed, but more optimistic about obtaining work after having reached a more reasonable size. I was at a weight where I felt ready to get back on the job market as a new, thinner me. That really should not have made a difference, but I thought I was more employable than I was at my presurgery weight.

Prior to leaving for Florida in December 2010, I was a bit stressed to get my home ready for Christmas and starting to eat badly. I was not eating the required protein, and sugar was creeping backing into my life. I was rewarding myself with chocolate—my worst temptation—and had headaches and felt bloated (a new feeling for me). Somehow the delusion that I could screw up in the short term and still make progress long term popped into my silly head. Not true!

The weight loss had opened many new doors for me and made me appreciate all the freedom it had returned to me. Before my surgery, I isolated myself and was fearful about being out in the world as my body expanded. After the surgery, I was looking forward to doing more and more as my body shrank. I wanted to play volleyball again and ride a bike. I felt more comfortable in social settings, and I owned how I felt in a more realistic manner. In the past I would not acknowledge my feelings of discomfort and put on a happy face, mentally counting down the minutes until the event was over. I went on vacation and then started counting down days to return instead of enjoying the moment. That mentality was due to my unhappiness about my weight and not being connected to my feelings.

Losing weight had improved the quality of my life but my relationships still needed work. The biggest relationship I had to manage was my relationship with myself. The pace of weight loss does change, and I had reached a plateau. The only way to continue to lose is to continue to eat healthy and up the activity level. So the work does not end, not ever!

When I was at my highest weight, I started a business that made jewelry for the plus-size woman and called it Big Bangles. Finding cool jewelry for a larger wrist, neck, or ankle was hard. I keep the business going for about four years, but beading became enormously popular and prices kept dropping until it became difficult to make a profit so I stopped altogether. Now I have to resize my own favorite jewelry!

I went to Florida again with Angela T. and we were even more active than the prior winter vacation—and I was able to keep up, even on the long walks Angela liked to take. I also worked out with her in the little gym where we were staying. I was not uncomfortable working out with another person, but I was not following the food plan much. I was doing my own thing, confident that the surgery would handle the rest. I was screwing around with my food—I was still thinking the old way of eating, just in smaller amounts.

Give Back

Hoping to help future patients, I had offered to rewrite the bariatric surgery orientation manual for the nurse coordinator. In a previous life, I was a technical trainer and wrote instruction guides in automotive, retail, banking, health care and more. I told the nurse coordinator that the manual was laid out in a confusing manner and that I thought I could improve on it if they would allow me to. She was willing to give me the file and work on it. No one in the department had the time or skills to work on it.

I restructured the manual by moving sections into a more logical sequence and putting the forms and check lists in the back as an appendix. I added some new material about the gastric sleeve procedure, since Henry Ford had just started offering it in 2009. This made the information flow better and follow the correct time sequence of pre-surgery, surgery, post-surgery activities. I felt that it would help future patients. I delivered the final copy in February 2011. I was still unemployed and thought it would be a kind service to those that had been so kind to me.

New Job

Early in 2011, things were still progressing with the weight loss. It was much slower. I was swimming two to three times a week at the Troy Community Center, trying to get to my goal: 250 pounds, my weight at high school graduation. That was not the surgical goal of 180 pounds end weight I was given. My appetite had waned, and I was not eating enough to stay healthy. I just didn't want to be bothered making meals or choices. I tried to maintain a routine but didn't quite make it through the week.

I received a job offer in February 2011 to work for Kelly Services (KellyOCG) as part of its engineering staffing division. I accepted it. The only downside to the position was that I would be working 100 percent from home. I really wanted to have the personal contact that came from working in an office, but this job was virtual. As with many business, Kelly was short of office space and trying new techniques of working with remote staff. My role was to recruit engineers for a Michigan-based company, Bosch.

I started work on March 6 and initially found the work easy, but the management structure was very confusing. There were a lot of bosses. We had weekly and daily status calls, and various people presented updates about their work.

Only 4 people worked on Michigan-based accounts, compared to the 18 or so who worked for clients elsewhere, so the calls were a good way for me to learn about my team and what they did.

Being back on the job added some structure to my life, but I was still struggling to reach my weight loss goal. Sitting at home on the computer or phone was a bit restrictive, and my restlessness led back to food. I still swam in the early mornings before work, and I thought that would help me continue to bring my weight down. But I started snacking to avoid the boredom of the job, and trigger foods crept back into the house. Before I knew it, I was back to eating chocolate, crackers, and snacks—junk food, not protein.

Food

Gastric bypass surgery created very real boundaries for my eating. I physically cannot eat as much as I did before, and I must eat slowly or I will vomit. These limitations prevent mindless consumption. I am forced to stay in the present and to be aware of what I am eating and how much. Getting sick—either vomiting or having diarrhea—has proved to be a great form of aversion therapy. Even if I wanted to eat a big cheeseburger or pizza, I know that doing so would make me ill, taking away any pleasure I might get. I still love certain smells: fresh pizza, hot rolls, a sizzling steak, but now my immediate response is to think that eating those things would make me sick, and that it is not worth it. Food no longer solves my problems the way it once did—or I thought it did.

From my teenage years to my early 40s, I thought eating provided comfort and escape from my stresses and anger. I stayed numb for a very long time. Once I started therapy and going to a 12-step program, I realized how much I was self-medicating. It took me a long time to take action and admit first that I was a food addict and second that I *had* to take action of some kind.

But even with those physical changes, the "monkey mind" of my food interactions came back. Monkey mind is when my thoughts swung back and forth between different choices or scenarios that I wanted to try to get what I wanted. I was unable to eat the foods or the amount of food that made every uncomfortable emotion go away. Instead, I had to deal with my feelings head on—which I was better equipped to do with the help of my therapist and a few close friends. I did not reach out for help much on the topic of my food addiction. Growing up it was such a double-edged sword. If I mentioned my problems to my family, I was met with little understanding or help other than that I should try another diet. I learned to not to go there for support. People in general did not understand food addiction; it was seen as lack of will power instead. I had a hard time accepting that it was considered a disease.

Instead of eating, I try to focus on what is pushing me to eat. Am I having a feeling of frustration that sends me to do laps in the kitchen, looking for something to eat for release? Once I identify the trigger, I deal with the trigger instead of eating mindlessly. I talk myself off of the ledge, as it were.

I learned to deal with issues quicker, and became more open to getting help and support from those around me. When something triggers me, I recognize the path of destruction for what it is, and my own sense of survival kicks in before I fall back into old patterns.

But even if I am better at denying it, my food addiction still exists, and it will never go away. I could easily fall back into old habits if I don't continue to understand and deal with my addictive behavior. Through treatment, counseling, and admitting that I am a food addict, I can understand what is going on in my head. I may be able to resist the cravings for a short time, but I will eventually give in. I spent my whole life knowing that certain foods calmed me, and for decades, I allowed myself to be calmed by them. But if I can understand the role food plays in my life, then perhaps I can change its role going forward.

Food

Have you noticed that "food" is a four-letter word?

Grocery Shopping

Grocery shopping is a real challenge. I still review the coupons from the newspaper and sometimes pull out a few for my past binge foods, and my food-obsessed mind will scheme about how I could consume them safely. (I liked to think that food I got on sale or for a "good deal" was worth eating no matter that it was bad for me.) But the pile of coupons is far smaller than it was in the past. I truly do stick to the outer aisles for grocery shopping—where the fresh, natural products are stocked—as is recommended by health professionals, because it is what I can safely eat and feel good about eating. I was spending less money on food too.

Even after years of binge eating and restricting, I never feel safe making food choices. I would do well for a while and then fall off the wagon and start making poor choices. Having the bariatric surgery did not correct my flawed thinking, so I still struggled with making the right choices even if I had limited eating capacity. You can still eat poorly after the surgery—you just eat less volume in one sitting. You can also graze all day long, and graze on bad food to boot. To have taken such a drastic step as having my stomach physically altered and then continue to eat poorly would be sabotaging myself—a potentially horrible outcome.

I hoped that the anger and frustration I had about how the surgery changed my relationship with food would subside and I would get past feeling cheated or restricted. The surgery itself was a minor inconvenience, but the change in food consumption was a hard lesson to process in my food addict's mind.

Variety is the key for me. I need to have choices, or I will get bored and start looking for inappropriate food. Cooking for one has always been hard, and the surgery made it even more challenging. It takes planning and concentration, which are things I always avoided when it came to food. I would not own my choices. So I need to have my cupboard stocked full and to always have an array of proteins, vegetables, and fruit to choose from. I have to avoid taking the easy way out—buying precooked meals, peanuts, cheese, eggs, etc.—and actually cook fresh, healthy, nutritious meals.

I used to eat a lot of fruit before surgery, but now that is lower on the list of good foods for me to have. Natural fruit has a lot of sugar in it. At the top of the list is protein, protein, and protein! But not just any kind of protein—I can't eat red meat, I can't eat pork, and I really miss meat. I miss the quantity of meat I used to eat. My older brother Peter ran a seafood restaurant for years, and after that he bought into an upscale steak house in Livonia, Michigan. I love to go there and eat a rib eye steak—or a New York strip, filet mignon, or lamb chops. But I couldn't for the first three to four years. Red meat was too dense for me to digest. Now I can eat small quantities of beef, very carefully. I miss my starches too—potatoes, pastas, breads, etc. They rank lower on the gastric food chain, not providing the protein or nutrients we need.

But even if he couldn't serve me a rib eye at his restaurant, Peter did the nicest thing one Christmas, years after I had the surgery. He and his wife served beef tenderloin but cooked a chicken breast for me! That was sooooo cool. Finally, my family was starting to get it. I never felt heard in the past about my food issues and the surgery seemed to tell the family that (1) I had a food problem, (2) I was serious about changing, (3) I was willing to discuss it, and (4) I was finally asking for help from them.

Binging

After about nine months after surgery, I went on many mini binges. Mostly eating mini candy bars—Butterfingers, Milky Ways, Dove chocolates, and others too. I would buy several bags of them (with a coupon or on sale of course) and treat myself. The problem is that I cannot pace myself when it comes to chocolate. Once I started, I would invariably finish the whole bag before the day was over—and sometimes I'd start in on a second bag as well. This lasted about three weeks. My weight loss declined and I had a persistent headache and felt horrible and uncomfortable. But once a food addict, always a food addict. It wasn't until I had realized and admitted that I had "relapsed" into old behavior and stalling the recovery process that I stopped fooling around with my food options.

I will be honest and say that I have had several relapses over the years. They've been shorter, and I recover more quickly now that I have greater of awareness and am in tune with my body and how it functions. But I know that dangerous path will always be one bite away.

Trying to eat like the old days is just not possible. Sometimes it's the quantity, and other times it's the type of food that triggers a bad reaction. Unfortunately I can still eat chocolate, much to my mother's dismay. (I remember that when I was being allergy tested my Mother said she hoped I turned up allergic to chocolate. No such luck.)

Emotional Eating (Monkey Mind)

I had a telephone argument with a family member who can be a bully and was unhappy with the call's outcome. I waited a while to see if the anger would pass and it did not. I called back that evening, and putting all my therapy to good use, I said: "I need to talk to you. These are my feelings and I want to say the following . . ." It was the first time I pushed back instead of holding on to the anger. Well, it did not go so well and we ended up hanging up on each other. Subsequently, we called each other back to apologize.

But I was still mad and upset and cried for a good hour and called another friend to bitch. The next day, I had errands to run, and one was stopping at the ACO Hardware store. I had a small list of items to get with coupons. It was also right before Christmas, and many items were already on sale: Christmas cards, decorations, paper products and CANDY. So after getting my coupon items, I headed toward the checkout and, lo and behold, there was the food aisle. And Christmas candy was 50 percent off! A sucker for bargains and especially food, I started putting things in my cart. Cheetos, cookies, candy, mints, and chips—I piled them all into my cart. When I finally checked out, I had four full bags, one of which was brimming with food.

I got home and began putting everything away except for the food. That food bag I left on the kitchen counter. When I was done putting everything else away, I grabbed a container of Cheetos and headed to the couch. I turned on the television and started to eat. After my third handful, I realized what I was doing. Man, I was mad. It was like being on autopilot. Bad or unpleasant feelings? Get food. Get food to stuff the feelings down. Eat food!

Awareness sucks. I took the Cheetos and dumped them down the garbage disposal. Then I looked at the rest of the food. I put it all back into the bag. I put the bag on the floor near the door. At first I was going to throw the food away. Over the next couple of hours, I experienced what I call "monkey mind" in the addiction business. Monkey mind is when an addict tries to figure a way to get what they want and rationalize it. I thought about getting rid of some of the food. I thought about spacing the food out over several days (hilarious, right?). I thought of about a million different scenarios to keep the food in the house. And then my sanity shouted above the din: TAKE THE FOOD BACK!

What a concept. Not only would I get it out of the house, I could get my money back too. Then stage 2 of monkey mind kicked in. I will take it back tomorrow, I told myself. I was already home and did not want to go out again. Mind you, this was about 2:30 in the afternoon and I had been home for three hours. I spent more time obsessing about the food: thinking about when to return it, thinking about whether I should return it at all. I was exhausted by 5:00 p.m. But I could not stand the emotional roller coaster, so I got into my car and returned everything. A breakthrough!

As a reminder to myself and how easy it is for me to tumble into the pit of eating, I took a picture of the pile of food. It's a picture that reminds me of the insanity my food addiction can cause even after bariatric surgery.

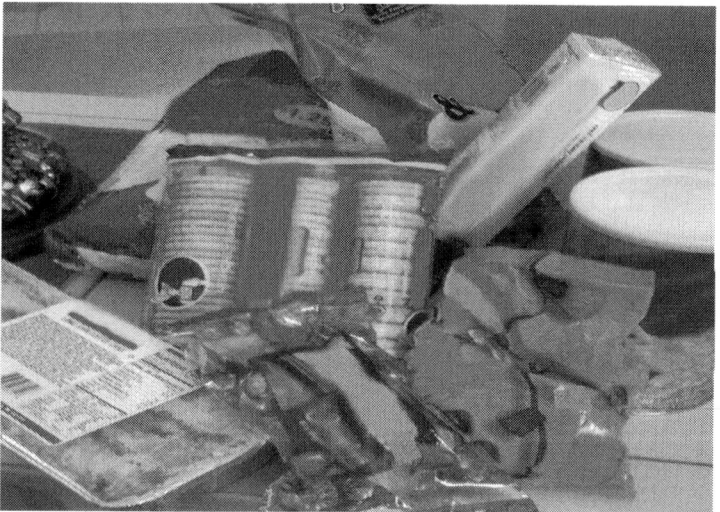

Now, the sad part is that in the past I would have polished this amount of food off in a day or two easily and not have cared.

Eating was a refuge for so long. When I ate, I felt safe and numb from any insecurities, fears, pain, frustration, or hopelessness. The numbness closed me off from the good feelings too, but for so long it seemed easier to live without those feelings and live with food. Before my surgery in 2009, I was slowly turning inward and could not see my future any longer. I wrote in my journal that year: "Luckily, I was going to therapy weekly and my great therapist reminded me that everything passes, think one day at a time and I could change if I wanted to do so."

Normalizing Food

What is normal eating? Can you define it? I sure can't. This is a discussion I have had with my therapist many times. It has been hard to wrap my head around this concept: normal eating. A few approaches were thrown out for discussion:

1. Eat well, and eat something really wonderful even if it is a small portion, which helps you appreciate the food more.

2. Since you're limited about what volume you can eat, make good choices.

3. Order what you want at a restaurant even if you don't finish it or want to take it home as leftovers. (Just because you had surgery, the denial method works only so long; then you cave.)

4. Ignore other people's expectations—they don't live in your body.

5. Food obsession does not disappear.

Money

Another component of eating for me is money. Yes, money. I have issues with money and food. I feel compelled to finish whatever food I purchase even if I know it's bad for me.

I think if I can get a deal like "two for one" or use a coupon or find a huge markdown, it is worth buying the food even if it is the wrong food. I hate to throw out food. I have so many rules about food in my head that I think it may explode. I ask myself, where do these mind games come from?

Mind Games

Throughout my life, I played mental games about food. Deciding when, what, and where to eat was always a major consideration. Do I eat before I go out to a social event in case I do not like the food? Should I stop at this drive-through on the way home or this other one? If I buy two for one, can I just eat the one and save the other? (Rarely.) With that history, how could I expect to deal with food after surgery in a rational manner? After all, I did not have brain surgery at the same time as the bariatric surgery.

So I still am learning. Trying to listen to my body when I eat and feel the "fullness"—the discomfort—telling me to stop. I rarely had digestive problems, which meant I could eat and eat and eat. But in learning to make better food decisions, and relearning food preparations skills, I realized that there is no real prize at the end of binge eating, that I hurt no one except myself.

Going out to eat is agonizing for me. First off, I want to eat something I don't cook at home. Then know that I will want to eat the leftovers; I don't want to waste money. Can I use a coupon? I can't beat the feeling that people are judging me either. And once I order something and the waiter brings it to the table, I have to eat slowly, and it is hard to go slow because for years I used to scarf food down before someone would take it away or suggest I had had enough. I still finish first and have to sit and watch others eat, which can be awkward for all unless we talk about it upfront and they are aware of my eating requirements. Finally, there is a lot of temptation to eat more and more to fill in the time.

Society emphasizes celebrating with food. Think of all the social occasions you attend: how many do not include food or drink? If I maintain friendships, must it be through dinning out or serving food? What happened to going for a walk or to the museum or playing cards—activities where the role of food is minimal, or where there is no food at all? We go to the bar after work, we have parties to celebrate milestones: graduation, births, divorces, new home, new job, or a death. Food is cheap and a common bond that people use to express their feelings and care for one another. So how does one do that without food?

Bariatric food suppliers offer a vast array of options. For the "right after" surgery patient, there are all kinds of protein shakes and recipes to adapt the powder protein into something edible. Further down the path, there are protein bars, cookies, treats, meals, snacks, drinks, and much more that are high in protein. And don't forget the vitamin and mineral supplements. These items are not cheap.

Ultimately, you need to eat real food. The protein shakes and supplements are a transition food. You're not meant to live on those for the rest of your life. People who have the surgery need to learn to make better choices from what is available. There were some patients who were afraid to start eating again and those who periodically return to the liquid protein to manage their weight.

How does one nourish herself and others without food?

Body Awareness

The changes in my body were hard to adapt to. Initially, changes happened pretty rapidly. And while getting recognition for the weight loss is a good thing, you have to remember I spent years thinking I was safe and hidden behind a wall of fat. Being more exposed or visible made me even more self-conscious during the transition.

Responding to comments on my weight loss made me uncomfortable at times and I had to come up with some phrases that normalized it for me. "I am a work in progress. Thanks for noticing. Thanks, it's a day at a time." People would comment on my neck, shoulder blades, hands, face, etc., like they were seeing them for the first time—and sometimes they were! Seeing the definition of my collarbone blows me away to this day. I don't remember being able to clearly see my collarbone since early childhood.

I did not notify a lot of people prior to my surgery because I was afraid I might chicken out, and I did not want to explain my decision over and over. After my surgery, I gained even more self-confidence after shedding some weight—not that I was ever lacking—and this changed the long-standing dynamics of several relationships. My friend Karen and I went shopping at a discount store once, and she remarked that she could not find me in the store. She said I blended in with the other people because I was within a more normal body size range. I took that as a compliment.

Body Changes

Every person's body reacts differently to weight loss. Age is a factor too. The elasticity of one's skin can be a determining factor in the approval process for future body contouring surgeries. As I have lost weight, I am slowly becoming more aware of my body and its flaws. Not to say I did not have them before—it was just that I learned to ignore them, pretend they did not exist. I used to think I hid them well with my clothing choices.

My new problem areas so far are what I call my "deflated" six-pack. My boobs, middle, and stomach failed to achieve a toned look and are sadly too wiggly for words. I hope to have at least a tummy tuck and an upper arm lift down the road. My first preferred surgery is definitely the tummy tuck because not only would it improve my appearance, it would remove some more weight. Bat wings, however, are priority number two. The upper arms did not snap back well and kind of flap around. I really would like to wear sleeveless tops or enjoy swimwear to the max.

Seeing my body clearly for the first time in a very long time was *scary*. I have to own it. I sure did not see it expand, so can I really see it shrink? As a woman, I would love to have all the surgical help possible, but I am not that big on pain. Hanging boobs are a common problem for women my age, so I can live with those. I could obsess about my body and feel self-loathing and hatred, but that serves no purpose. After years of ignoring my body, I cannot beat it up for lack of self-care.

Certainly weight loss can improve your self-esteem; it can

change your personality as you get more comfortable being in public and more mobile. I know during my ongoing weight loss I felt more confident. I approached different physical activities that I avoided before with hopefulness. My stamina, breathing, and coordination was better as well as my attitude. I am open to new challenges and adventures like working out regularly and walking now that I feel I fit in better physically.

But that can be a problem for some people, especially if a recovering patient is leaving a spouse behind as they spread their wings, so to speak. In a support meeting, one patient mentioned that her husband was sabotaging her efforts to lose weight by bringing home treats and trigger foods she was finding it hard to resist. The psychologist said that this was not uncommon. I noticed that as I lost my initial 75 pounds, not much changed, but as I crossed over the 125-pound mark some of my heavier friends became less supportive and wondered aloud why I bothered to have the surgery.

Body Acceptance

Weight loss is an incredibly personal issue. And if you have issues before surgery, you will probably have the same issues after surgery unless you get help. I had a lot of shame, guilt, and self-loathing as I gained weight. I also had a lot of anger, arrogance, and attitude that I built up to protect myself from feeling rejected, unwanted, unloved, and out of control. I certainly did not turn those feeling off once the pounds started melting. In a sense, my weight was a garment that I shielded my body in, hoping no one would see me. But secretly, I wanted to be rescued.

Jewelry

Like nearly all parts of my body, my fingers are now smaller, and my ring size has dropped. I can wear some of my older rings that I had set aside from when I was younger and smaller in size.

Skin

Skin is much more noticeable when it is sagging than when it is fat. My skin was fairly firm when I was at my heaviest—it was stretched to the maximum and did not jiggle too much. However, as I have lost weight, the sagginess of my skin became pronounced. My arms and stomach truly sag now. Skin texture changes as well. And the older you are, the less resilient your skin becomes. It will not spring back to a smooth line. Right now, my arms look like cheesy bat wings— ugh. But I will take that look over still having the excessive weight and the promise of a shorter lifespan.

My remaining weight is primarily in my stomach and middle, and it will be hard to lose the belly fat, but I will keep working at it the best I can. I never really liked my body before and now the trouble spots seem more pronounced. But I really think it is because I am more present with myself, more connected to my feelings, and willing to look at all aspects of my life that I am so body aware. I never really looked at my body and did not notice when I gained weight unless I had to buy new clothes. I did not own my body. I may have inhabited it, but I was not connected to it. If I could check out mentally, then I did not have to take care of my body physically it either.

Feet

My feet are becoming less calloused; the skin is softer, and so I don't have to go the foot doctor every six weeks or so to get rid my calluses. My feet were really being punished by the excess weight. Now, I can go every two to three months! I can save money. My feet are about a half shoe size smaller too and don't swell daily anymore.

Vision Issues

I had some potentially dangerous vision issues before my surgery, which have cleared up due to the weight loss. Weight adds pressure all over, including in the eyes. My left eye wept—it was always tearing. I had some small hemorrhages in my left eye, and at first, the retinal doctor felt it was due to high blood pressure or diabetes, but I did not have either disease. These were definitely warning signs of what might have lain ahead if unchecked. There was a possibility of losing my sight in that eye. But after I had lost about 70 pounds, my test results at the retinal doctor were much improved, and at 160 pounds below my presurgery weight, the problems disappeared altogether. Once again I can save money because I only have to go once a year to see the retina specialist.

Hair

The surgery did a number on my hair—or rather to my body's ability to absorb calcium, which affects hair. I always had fine, thick curly hair before the operation. I could wash my hair and finger-dry it and it would look cute. Now the *curl is gone*, and my hair has thinned quite a bit, especially in the front. Hair loss is a common side effect of this surgery. So I went to a much shorter hairstyle to compensate. My hair requires more help in the mornings to get a manageable look rather than staying flat and tired.

Aches and Pains

My body and bones ached a lot during the first year after my operation, and I believe this also had to do with calcium. With a smaller stomach, bariatric patients have a more difficult time maintaining sufficient levels of the nutrient—and being depleted causes all sorts of odd things to occur. So I highly recommend you adhere to the guidelines from your doctor. My family and friends can attest that before the surgery I was never cold, but afterward, I was constantly freezing. This sensitivity can be linked to malnourishment and/or vitamin and calcium deficiencies. My sensitivity has lessened now, and oddly enough, my legs are rarely cold.

Medication

There are lots of pills to take after the surgery. Depending on the type of surgery and how the patient responds to it, vitamins (particularly B_{12}), calcium, and other supplements may be necessary. I have two other medications I need to take daily: a thyroid pill and an anti-anxiety medication, but I have noticed that they do not work the same as before the surgery. After discussion with my internal medicine doctor, we determined that my stomach did not absorb them the way they used to, so I needed to space them out so they would be effective again. My digestive system is different, and I have to adjust certain elements of my life around it.

The vitamin and calcium supplements are large in size, and I have to cut them up to swallow them safely. If I take the supplements with liquid, I have to plan around my food schedule. It is extremely uncomfortable and sometime impossible to eat and drink at the same time. With a stomach that can only hold three to four ounces of any substance, it is usually one or the other (food or liquid) with a minimum of 30 minutes in between. Timing is important for eating, drinking, and pill taking alike. I take the lowest amount of medications compared to many other gastric bypass patients, which is not good for me. I could have an adverse reaction or be sick if the timing is off. Like any addict, I can too easily ignore what my body needs to be healthy, supplements included. If I don't follow the guidelines, my body will suffer and the gastric tool will be broken.

Exercise

My entrance back into exercise took the form of water aerobics. I just love the water, so the pool was a logical place for me to turn. I started off slow, exercising twice a week at the community center, and then built up to three of four times a week. I felt great and was pleased with the progress. I was comfortable going into the pool as my body continued to change. My after-surgery routine was working and I liked the results.

Rewards

About a year into the weight loss, around November 2010, I became comfortable with my new life. I had learned how to eat out with friends and family and had more energy and stamina than I had felt in years—maybe decades. That fall, I went on vacation to England to see my brother John and his wife, Kate. I was thrilled that I was able to walk and see the sites without difficulty breathing, walking, and talking. My comfort level flying overseas was greatly improved. I did not have to upgrade to feel comfortable in the seat, nor did I need a seat belt extender. Compared to the trip I took in 2007, before the surgery, the vacation was pure fun!

It was the same way when I went to Florida for the holidays in 2011. I was more energetic and eager to visit tourist sites and walk around. I could really enjoy my time there.

Balance Issues

Learning to walk again has been a challenge. Between the weight loss and my falls, I felt I was walking off-center. I tended to stumble and forget to lift my feet up. I am very cautious on steps and uneven surfaces. My center of gravity has changed after the surgery, and I had to adjust to the new distribution of my weight as the pounds came off.

But another upside of the weight loss is that I can cross my legs. Now, you may think that is not a big deal—but put a pillow between your legs and then try to cross them and you will see what I had been dealing with. Crossing my legs makes me feel incredibly *girly*.

In December 2010, I wrenched my back, and my orthopedic doctor suggested physical therapy, core strengthening, and working to improve my balance. I was nervous about walking, since I had fallen twice. But the doctor said the therapy should help improve my balance and gait. During the process, I started using long-dormant muscles and breaking up the stiffness of arthritis that occurred over the years. It really helped me gain a broader range of motion.

I started a five-week stint of physical therapy after my fall in February 2010, and I soon began feeling a lot of pain in my back and left knee. I was worried I had done some harm, so I went to my orthopedic surgeon for a conversation and X-rays. His review said I had hurt myself. The X-rays also showed a lot of arthritis in my joints, and the doctor laid out my options: I could do physical therapy and take anti-inflammatory drugs, take steroids, or have surgery. I opted for the first choice.

On the advice of my "new age" neighbor Sharon, I contacted Neil King at the physical therapy center in Rochester Hills, Michigan, to arrange for treatment. It was not a traditional practice. My hour of physical therapy treatment consisted of a half hour of stretches and exercises and a half hour of "Rolfing"—or stretching the muscle, tissue, and tendons. It was like a mini massage but much more intense. Rolfing was part of the treatment. (Rolfing is a process of organizing and lengthening the connective tissue in the body so that it relates with ease in gravity, giving muscles the space to move and joints the freedom to function.)

I did two treatments a week for five weeks. After the third session, I noticed when I was lying on my left side in bed that there was minimal pain in my knee. Previously, I had stopped lying on my left side because the knee would hurt and throb too much when it touched the mattress. Improvement already—so great!

Part of my discussion with the physical therapist was that I felt unbalanced at times and that with my weight loss, my center of gravity or my depth perception was off. He agreed that could be the case and said I needed to relearn how to walk. One method was to place my heel down first when I walk, then lean into the toes to push off. I realize that I had been dragging my feet, leading with my toes, and it caused me to shuffle. After just four sessions and a bit of at-home exercise, I could tell a difference.

I purchased some weights that can be worn on the wrists

or ankles to use at home. The remainder of the sessions focused on strengthening muscles and getting better balance. I have exercises to practice at home and hope I will continue to improve on all levels. As a much heavier person, I did not use a lot of my muscles and now have to strengthen them to make them work with my far lighter body. I want to be limber enough to go back to old hobbies and sports like volleyball and bike riding that physically challenged me even at my healthiest.

The evaluation after 30 days showed significant improvement in my range of motion. I was able to extend physical therapy for two more weeks. In the end, I felt much more comfortable with my body and balance. It was well worth it. It was April by then, and I was looking forward to spring so that I could walk outside and soak up the sunshine. In the meantime, I continued my swimming and exercises.

Mom

In July 2011, my mother, Kay, had a fire in her condo. She, of course, waited a day to tell me what happened. I rushed to her home, where I found there was smoke damage caused by her iron catching the ironing board on fire. She doused the fire with water and thought she could handle the cleanup. My mother was 85 years old at the time, and tiny. I told her she could not stay at home and had to come stay with me. So I moved her into my house and called the insurance company. I did not call my brothers for help. I did not run this by my therapist. I just reacted. Not the best choice on my part.

The insurance company started cleaning the condo top to bottom and checking for any electrical damage. The whole placed was cleaned: walls, furniture, clothing, cupboards, etc. The process took about a month and the bill was just under $40,000. At this time, the condo was not worth that amount due to the faltering Michigan economy.

During the month my mother stayed with me, I realizef she was much frailer. She did not eat much, and at five foot three she weighed just 100 pounds. I decided she should stay with me and sell the condo; once again, I did not consult my brothers, and I did not talk to my therapist. I took charge. I was making decisions, and my mother let me do so. Neither of us really discussed this decision or included other family members. I think my mother was a little scared and tired and glad that I took over. It also seemed she was happy not to be alone. My mother never spoke about her feelings; she always appeared independent and not reliant on anyone else, something she tried to instill in her children. That was a detriment because we chose not ask for help when it was available, leaving us frustrated and stressed.

Once my mother got settled, she started to assert herself and started to nag me about the condo, living arrangements, and insurance issues. My Aunt Melba came to visit and mediate between my mother and me. We bitched and screamed at each other for a few hours. My mother, Kay, conceded she should not live alone, so we decided to sell the condo and move her stuff to my house. She did not want to give up her independence but realized she needed help. Her hearing had diminished 50 percent, and her strength was diminished so she required help with chores, cleaning, and groceries. I packed up her belongings and either sold or donated the furniture. I had to add shelving in my basement to hold her pantry items and duplicate kitchen gear. All the while this was happening, my childhood fantasy of having a nurturing mother came to the surface. I thought we could reconnect and be different. Why I thought things would be different, I have no clue. But the child in me wanted Mom!

My mother really settled in. She positioned her chair to have a direct view of the television; her side table, knick-knacks, snacks, and cigarettes took over the living room. Her newspapers and books occupied a corner of the living room, the radio nearby.

And with her in the house, I struggled to stay centered and on my food plan. After just four months of living with her, I had gained 18 pounds. While my mother did not have an eating problem, she liked to nibble. She would have different jars of candy and cookies just in case she wanted to eat a bite. Needless to say, my hands strayed often to her containers.

On weekdays, I usually worked in the kitchen instead of my spare-bedroom office. I liked being able to look outside and walk around, take a break, get something to eat, and read the newspaper for a bit. Stuff like that. Well, that did not work so well anymore. Mom was always asking what I was doing from her recliner in the living room. She thought when I was on the phone, I was talking to her, and she would interrupt me when she had questions. I had to retreat upstairs.

I ate.

I made bad food choices.

At 85, my mother had pretty much stopped cooking. She typically went out to eat every other day and ate the leftovers as her next-day meal. So I was trying to cook healthy for myself but had to include my mother's needs as well. She always wanted to go out to eat. She would offer to pay to make it easier on me (supposedly).

We tried to compromise but it did not go well. I was slowly gaining my weight back. I had tried to keep swimming in the mornings, but that routine was cracking. My mother had numerous treats around, so there was always something for her to nibble on. She needed to gain weight. These jars called my name, and I often helped myself to them, grabbing a handful of candy or a couple of cookies. It got so bad that I would have to buy replacement items so my mother would not notice my eating habits.

Tension mounted as my mother and I began to bicker. We had a long history of bickering and fighting. We criticized one another, with one of us saying the other was not doing things the "right" way. I started to get resentful. My mother had pretty much taken over the first floor. I had to install a TV in my bedroom (something I had never done before) because to watch TV, I had to do it elsewhere. My mother took control of the remote and the first-floor TV.

I hated being upstairs all day and now at night. I started eating in my bedroom. Also another first.

I conferred with my Aunt Melba and arranged for my mother to visit her for a few days to give me a break. Mom was resistant but we persuaded her in the end. We worked out a routine where she would visit my Aunt Melba in Onsted, Michigan (90 miles away) about every six weeks for a couple of days. I needed this space.

I was stressed. I was resentful. I was angry. And I had no one to blame but myself. Therapy continued and my therapist strongly recommended that my mother should go to a senior residence. I felt like I would be a failure if I could not take care of her at this stage of her life. I struggled with the idea of telling my mother to leave.

I was an emotional wreck. I was no longer putting myself first and taking care of my eating, physical activity, or any recovery effort. All of the routines I had worked to establish quickly disappeared. I resorted to food. Six months after she moved in, my weight was up to 312. I had gained 50 pounds.

Vacation and Realization

Around this time, I planned a two-week vacation with my mother, Kay, and Aunt Melba to Florida for late February and March 2012. I thought that it would be a nice change of pace, and the two ladies could entertain each other and allow me some free time. I thought this would be a nice adventure, since I did not know if my mother would be able to travel in the future, and at the time, she seemed good to go.

I rented a cottage in Jensen Beach, Florida, so that we could have our own space, cook if we wanted to, and avoid the confusion of hotel guests. The first week went great. We explored, saw the sights, shopped, and hung out. The weather was wonderful.

The second week, the weather got cooler and wetter. The ladies got crabby. I got frustrated. When I got groceries, I was buying cookies and chocolate for myself, and sneaking them into my bedroom. I hid the wrappers or included them in other packaging to disguise them. My eating was out of control. My emotions and stress level were off kilter. I could no longer deal with the dynamics between my mother and myself. I was crying myself to sleep.

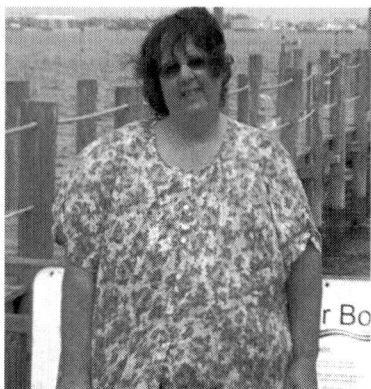

March 2012

I knew when we got home something had to change—but I was so scared to think of what that change might be, I ate *more*! With my therapist's encouragement, I called my brothers and told them I was stressed to the max and could no longer keep Mom with me. I cried through the phone calls. But my brothers offered support and asked what I needed. I didn't quite trust that they would help but they did.

John, my youngest brother, came in and helped me a lot. In many ways, John was like Switzerland when it came to my mother. He was neutral in that he had little interaction with her and when it occurred, everyone involved was on their best behavior. John and his wife usually visited once in the summer and again at the Christmas holidays. John was my sounding board as far as my mother was concerned. I did not have same the relationship with my two older brothers, Paul and Peter. They pretty much ignored my challenges with Mom.

John was able to persuade my mother to look at different senior residences and talked to her about what was the best situation for all involved. He tried to represent both sides fairly without emotions clouding the issues, something that was hard for me to do.

My mother gave me the silent treatment after I told her that I could no longer handle the living arrangements and she had to move out. Then she moved on to being angry with me. She said I had forced her to move into my home in the first place. I forced her to sell her condo. I was the bossy one. I upset her life. I changed everything for no good reason. She told me that my life had been out of control since long before the fire.

As much as I could, I explained to her that it was not about her directly but how I felt being with her and how I felt an outsider in my home. I didn't outgrow the early dynamics of childhood. We had had several conversations over the previous months and had actually grown closer. But this issue of my discomfort was foreign to my mother. Emotions were not something my mother dealt with—she was more of a fact-based person.

John and I took my mother to visit five different facilities. She ended up picking one, Pine Ridge of Garfield, that I had originally looked at several months earlier when we were discussing options. It was two miles from her previous home, a familiar setting that reassured her, close to her friends, shopping, movies, the library, and more. The apartment she chose had its own kitchen, two bathrooms, a bedroom, lots of storage, a parking spot, and an outside entrance as well as an internal one. Meals and laundry were provided as part of the rent but she could cook if she wanted to. Each day, they asked that she notify them she was up by hitting a button; otherwise she was free to do as she wanted. She moved in April 2012.

Brothers Paul, Peter, and John and grandson Andrew helped with the move. We also arranged for Paul to stay with her the first two nights. She settled in fairly well. After the first week, I saw a small change in her attitude toward me and a cheerfulness. She had discovered pinochle night and the facility van would take her to the library, shopping, or doctors. My mother also thought she would be the oldest person there and was surprised to find several women older than her at the dining table.

I was worried that my brothers would think less of me since I could not take care of our mother. They never said that to me. It was all my projections on them. I felt so relieved that we were taking action. I did not have to do this by myself. And I got my home back. My food intake started improving within a week. I started sleeping better. I reached out to people in my 12-step program. I was trying to stay in the present.

I visited her often in the beginning, two to three times a week. I still took her to doctor's visits and drove her van to keep it working. By the third week, we chatted and she surprised me by saying she was really enjoying the residence. It offered her people in her age bracket, outings of interest, lots of activities, and good meals when she wanted. I was relieved she seemed happy and content with the decision. The strain between us was lightening. I was reclaiming my home and sanity.

The fourth week, I took my mom to the doctor's on Tuesday. She got a clean bill of health for her age and had gained some weight. The doctor was pleased and all was good. Wednesday, I called her before her 6:30 p.m. card group to chat and said good night. Brother John called after 9:00 p.m. to tell her that he and his wife had bid on a new house and chatted for a while.

Childhood Relationships

Family

My mother never asked me much about my feelings, but as I have gone through this weight loss journey, I've tried to explain its impact on my life. I had trained her over the years *not* to ask me about my weight or how I felt, and it's hard to open that door up. But I tried to share my changes with her, the little victories and milestones that brought out how the change had helped my overall health and outlook on life. (My mother was slender, usually a size 8 or 10, never larger than a size 12.) These discussions provoked some interesting questions between the two of us.

Our overall relationship was always rocky. My mother was not a demonstrative person; connection was made by actions, doing rather than being. She rarely held my hand, hugged me, or touched me. I related to her what I did or what I was going to do. Our relationship was measured a success by what we did for others, family, and work. My three brothers have shared different levels of interest. My two older brothers, Paul and Peter, have always been tall and slender and we did not interact much growing up. My youngest brother, John (13 years younger), and I share more of the same body characteristics and weight issues. These we get from my father's side of the family.

Both sides of my family have serious health issues. On my mother's side was heart disease and high blood pressure. Father's side had arthritis, diabetes, and weight issues.

Although I was a "preemie," I soon became a chubby little girl. I don't know why. I was described as "sturdy," "husky," and "chubby." Which was not exactly fun!

Bariatric surgery *can* put stress on relationships. I could put unrealistic expectations on myself and others as far as my progress and expect people to treat me better now that I was out in the open about my food. Get love and acceptance where it did not occur before with friends and men. I resisted family and friends' attempts to help, as I saw myself as being independent and private. Both before and after surgery I worried that people would sabotage me by offering foods that were inappropriate. After I had gone to a rehab facility for food addiction in 2001 for 45 days, people tried to serve me items I had identified as trigger foods, and in less than two months, I started falling back into my old unhealthy habits.

I had to find new ways to connect, socialize, and celebrate without over focusing on foods. As the Henry Ford Bariatric Center suggests to friends and families in its orientation manual:

1. Learn as much as you can about bariatric surgery.

2. Attend as many educational classes, doctor visits and support groups as you can.

3. Recognize this surgery as physically and emotionally stressful. Your loved one has to re-learn to eat and to change lifelong patterns with food. Be thoughtful of the food you bring into the hospital room and your home as your family member(s) adjust to these changes.

4. Don't become the "food police" and monitor everything your loved one is eating and not eating. However, if you

notice that your loved one is straying from his/her medical recommendations, mention that you are concerned about his/her behavior and ask what you can do to help.

5. Recognize your own feelings of anger, resentment or fear. Talk with your loved one about these feelings and find others who may share your experience.

6. If relationships become stressed, seek out counseling to help you both adjust to these new changes in your life.

The manual further states:

Some people, including family and friends of a person with life-long obesity may not understand the true nature of obesity. It is a disease with many factors involved including genetic, social, psychological, environmental and medical. Even people who support you and have witnessed your struggles with weight through the years may not understand that obesity is a disease and is not simply a matter of no will power and lack of self-control. Having this belief, they may feel that by considering obesity surgery, you are "taking the easy way out." With time and seeing your long-term success with your weight and healthier lifestyle, their understanding and support should grow.

Betrayal

As I entered the workforce in my early years, I aligned myself with other plump individuals. We could be comfortable eating and socializing together, and it helped diminish the stares and other less obvious forms of discrimination and judgment. But once you were part of the group, you were not supposed to change. I have several chubby friends who have known me for more than 20 years. We tended to travel, shop, and eat together, and initially my chubby friends were very supportive, but as my weight loss became noticeable, their attitudes changed. Originally, I was the largest of the group, but as I approached their respective sizes and then went below them, they became cranky.

In my journal, I wrote that I watched my friends eat and eat, and I whined a little to myself. Yes, I wanted to eat that whole package of donuts, cookies, candies, etc., but my body rebelled and the rebellion hurt worse than the desire to eat. If I went out to a meal with friends, I realized I held judgment about their choices. I felt that if I had to be restricted so should they, no matter what size they were—silly, right? I wanted them to notice and compliment me on my sacrifices so I could feel better about myself and the choices I made in having the surgery. However, after advising them it was okay to eat in front of me during my transition, it became difficult for me to watch them eat. No one really noticed what I ate, only if I didn't eat.

When we went to dinner, which I did less of because (1) I could not eat as much, (2) I could not afford it, as I was not working, and (3) what I got typically gave me two to three days of leftovers, I would ordered just one item while the others would order drinks, an appetizer and/or salad, main entrée, dessert, and coffee. Since I can't eat more than three or four ounces at a time, I would finish sooner than the rest. (I am a cheap date.) When I was through eating, I could still carry on the conversation.

Over time, the invitations to dinner from my chubby friends came less and less frequently, which was sad; I never discussed what we were eating or passed judgment on them because I was addressing my own issues with food. I guess they felt uncomfortable around me. So instead of celebrating my success, my chubby friends have fallen by the wayside, while most of my healthy-sized friends have been great cheer-leaders. They see the benefits of my actions and are supportive and encouraging.

Dating

I did not date much in high school. I dated a bit in college. As a chubby woman, I was not the first one the males I met wanted to date. I was "the buddy," the "funny one," and the "organizer" in the group.

My dating life improved when I started working. I had more confidence and took the role of the seeker. There were singles booklets with ads for men and women seeking to date and some specialized in men who liked bigger women. That made it a bit more likely I would be chosen. Letters were sent through a service and if there was interest, you met. I met a few men but had no long-term relationships.

When the Internet blossomed, I joined online dating sites that featured men who liked the "larger" ladies (BBW Lovers, BBW Dating, Linda's Social Club, etc.). Even on these sites, men were still discriminating in their criteria: preferring a big stomach, big boobs, big ankles, a pear-shaped body, "junk in the trunk," and so on. But at least I felt there was more chance of meeting someone who was comfortable with my overall large physical appearance and wanted to be with me. I was definitely a "pear."

I meet many men and oddly found some who said I wasn't big enough. How crazy is that? I met a lot of men. Unfortunately, many were also married (not interested) or just wanted sex (again, not interested). Men feel that if you are overweight you will settle for anything or do anything. Not this woman! Dating as a plus size is just as difficult as being in a normal range.

I dated off and on for years but I almost never shared that information with family and friends. First, I was always insecure about the relationship and how long it might last. Second, sometimes the men I picked were not ones I wanted to introduce to my world. The underlying feelings I had dating and having relationships was shame. Shame that I was not good enough. Shame that my body was fat, and who could love or even like a body like mine? Shame that this person who liked me could like someone so fat.

Luckily my attitude did mature and the shame lessened. I was fortunate to meet some really nice men in my later 40s and early 50s that I spent time with and grew to care about. But I never introduced them to family. My longest relationship with a BBW (Big Beautiful Woman) lover was four years and he passed away with cancer in December 2007. He loved my size, and if I lost weight, he noticed and commented that it looked like I had lost weight. "You are not as fluffy. What are you doing?" Only a few friends met him. None of my family except John, my younger brother, knew about him.

I also blame myself for not being comfortable in relation-ships. I did not accept for a long time that some men preferred larger ladies. I thought they were odd. I know better now. It's sad that I compartmentalized my life in order to cope, but that was how I coped. In therapy, I was learning to integrate all the parts of my life, but old habits die hard. I still wasn't letting people close while I was on this journey. Bariatric surgery changed some of that. As I lost weight, I tried to describe to my family what the changes were doing to me emotionally and physically. Some were interested, while others were not. But as I said earlier, surgery gave me verbal diarrhea—I needed to talk.

I spent a lot more time talking to my mother. I was finally willing to discuss how I had felt the many years prior to my surgery and how "fat" affected me. We had some very candid conversations. I was able to tell her how I felt when she took me to doctors, Weight Watchers and TOPS as a child. I spoke to the fact that her comments were always about what I should be doing, not acknowledging what I was doing or how well. We took baby steps. Kay admitted that she did not know what to do and did the best she could in this area, as she never had a weight problem. She did not understand how damaging it was to a young child to be treated like a "defective object"—my words, not hers. The more willing I was to talk, the more cautiously she asked questions. And considering how I used to respond (with anger, abruptness, the silent treatment), it was a big improvement in our overall relationship.

12-Step Program

I joined a 12-step program almost 15 years ago when I first got serious about recognizing my problem. I had gone to a treatment facility for eating disorders in 2001. Participating in a 12-step program was required as part of follow-through after leaving treatment. Even after 45 days at a rehab facility, I still didn't get it. It was still too new for me to get and keep recovery.

12-step program membership helped me understand that food addiction and compulsive eating is an illness. You can be rational and capable of working and raising a family and be a great volunteer and a consistent spiritual person, but when it comes to food—insanity rules! My 12-step program experience opened my eyes to what the illness is and what forms it takes in different people. And how difficult (with a low success rate) the program of abstinence is. In a 12-step program, abstinence is defined as not eating compulsively whether you are overweight, anorexic, or bulimic.

Gastric bypass surgery was viewed as "cheating" by some 12-step program members. Some thought if you worked the program hard enough you would not need surgery. You could resolve your weight issues through the program alone. I was not one of those people. Those in the 12-step program who had strong recovery could be a little judgmental. In fact, gastric bypass surgery was never a topic at a meeting, retreat, or open talk. I did not broadcast my surgery but if people asked I would tell them what I had done. As some of the 12-step program members found out, several shared with me that they had gone that route but kept quiet at meetings.

I remember in 2006 two men coming to the 12-step program who had had the surgery but gained their weight back, and I thought, how sad. But they worked the program and I knew at least one who has attained his goal weight again. That is a daily reminder to me of what could happen to me if I don't use all the tools available to me both with the 12-step program (plan of eating, writing, meetings, reaching out through telephone calls, etc.) and without (support groups, websites, etc.).

Neighbors

For some neighbors, my weight loss deepened friendships and others just ask general questions about it. Most are happy with my success. I have attempted to expand those friendships by going walking with them so that I keep my activity level up and discover new outlets of fun. I stay connected and continue to exercise my evolving shape. Oddly, some neighbors are warmer toward me now that I have lost the weight. Maybe I am more relatable and approachable as well as less defensive. I was really very unhappy in my fat state for a long time, and it probably showed in my attitude.

I love to swim and have a pool at my complex. Whenever possible in the summer months, I love to relax by the pool and see my neighbors. Friends visit; we hit the pool, then shop and/or dine. This made me realize that I need to cultivate more active friends in general, and as a result of this past summer, two neighbors, two newer friends and I signed up for evening water aerobics at the Troy Community Center for 4 months.

My Mother's Passing

Thursday at 7:00 a.m., I get a call from the senior residence, Pine Ridge, stating that my mother was taken to the hospital by ambulance at 4:00 a.m., but she insisted that they not call me till 7:00 a.m. so I would have a good night's sleep. I rushed to the hospital. She was in cardiac care because her heart was beating irregularly. Something else was going on and they were doing tests. I reached out initially to my brother Peter, who lived locally.

As time went on, we learned that she had a blocked bowel. Due to the fact she had emphysema and a heart condition, she was not a candidate for surgery. This basically was a death sentence. There was nothing to be done. I was devastated. I thought about all that had transpired in the last month and thought that somehow I had caused this problem. I sought food to numb out.

The family came in. It was Mother's Day weekend and the grandkids were in town. Everyone got to visit with Mom during these last few days. She passed on the following Wednesday. While I had been on track mending our relationship, I felt I lost out on forging a new healthier relationship with my mother.

I was a wreck. I took time off work. My brothers stayed a few days and we decided to hold a memorial service later in the summer so we could honor our mother properly. I said goodbye to them and then had to deal with the aftermath. I had to coordinate the cremation, deal with the cemetery, handle the notices, accounts, doctors, bills, etc. Once again, I arranged for movers to transport her possessions back to my home, all the while using food to handle my distress and the emotional roller coaster. Surgery did not prevent my abuse of food during this time.

The memorial service was in July and the family gathered. It was a respectful and pleasant event with family and good friends. I was happy at how it turned out and felt that we had closure and honored my mother properly.

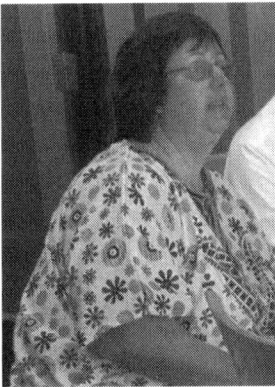

July 2012

After my mother's death in May 2012, I really struggled with food and emotions. I felt that I had let her down and that I was a "bad daughter" even though I knew it was not true. But it was how I felt. And those feelings made me eat. It was hard to have closure with her because of her unexpected death.

I still had to work daily and deal with closing my mother's estate, moving her possessions, and the daily correspondence. I did not ask for help. I thought it was my duty to do it all. I never considered that my brothers might or might not want to help me.

I created a spreadsheet and monitored all the activity so I had proof to my brothers that all was handled fairly. I wrote the letters, responded to inquiries, closed credit cards, sold furniture, made donations, etc. My emotions were sometimes nonexistent and other days all over the place. I could not get a grip on my eating either. Dove chocolates became my go-to coping food. They were small, went down easy and made me mellow. And they were frequently on sale.

Those activities kept those negative feelings in front of me daily. I started eating the wrong foods, grazing during the day. (I worked from home so food access was easy.) Totally ignoring what I was doing to myself. I was going to therapy but words were not penetrating the food fog. I also kept obsessing about what could have been done differently while knowing that there really had been no other choices. I was over-thinking and overreacting, totally forgetting what years of therapy and my 12-step program had taught me. I just did not care enough about myself to stop eating.

Laid Off

Just as I was finally coming out of the food fog, I got laid off on Monday, October 1, 2012. I remember it well, as I got a call around 11:00 a.m. from my boss saying that I was laid off and to stop working. It was a shock! Business had been slow and they had been moving our team around to other accounts as needed. It pulled any stability out of from under me, another routine disrupted.

Now I was grieving and unemployed and knew it was unlikely I would find a job in the fourth quarter; I turned to food again, which was cheap, accessible, and silent. I had not resumed swimming at the Troy Community Center in the mornings. I could not get traction on my eating or exercising. I had been unemployed before. This time I took it a lot harder. I was an older and experienced candidate and that made it more difficult to be hired in the current Detroit market. I think I was feeling detached from the world and couldn't see my next steps.

Therapy became very important because I had always had issues with my mother and now with her gone, there was no opportunity for resolution. My unresolved issues list got a little longer. Oddly enough, there was a shift in the burden/obligation I had always felt toward my mother. It was a crazy mix of emotions. Emotions made me ravenous. I ate. I was regaining the weight I had lost. Poor eating, no exercise, and limited social activities were eroding the progress I had made in the first year and half after surgery.

This is where I felt that the medical community failed me after surgery. Yes, surgery was successful. Yes, I lost weight. Yes, I changed my eating habits—for a while. But the ultimate component in the recovery was changing my thinking. Surgery did not do that. I think I thought for a brief moment that it would. I found out differently. There were sessions on nutrition, what to eat, how often to eat, the need to eat a certain way, but not on how to change the obsessive thinking about food and the way I interacted with food. Here I thought the surgery would be the cure-all and I would be strong enough to avoid gaining the weight back. SURPRISE! Not true. I had not truly changed my personal food thinking or behavior.

While I still had some items I could not eat (bacon, steak, pork, etc.) I was able to resume eating many of the foods I enjoyed previously but in smaller portions (pizza, bread, cheese, etc.). Once my fear of eating subsided, I resumed eating many of the same foods that got me into trouble before. Not surprisingly, I continued to gain weight.

Here I was, eating unhealthy, fat, sugary foods again—though slower—not exercising, isolating (not attending 12-step program meetings or socializing with friends) and being shut down emotionally. This mode of behavior continued through the winter and into early 2013. I started to recover from my emotional bottom in late spring of 2013. I had dealt with most of my mother's affairs and felt that there was some light ahead. I was aware that I had regressed socially and was anxious to get out and about again. There was a light ahead of me and in me. I was relieved to get back on track and into some kind of routine.

Obsessive Behavior

I am a person who seeks help but will not always take it. I have been in therapy a long time and can easily tell you that I have had the same conversations for many years with my therapist about eating and how I cannot stay on a diet. How I can't commit to writing my food down. How no one understands what I am going through. How no one feels the way I do. Which was all my bullshit, or so I tried to convince myself. If I had no feelings, I did not exist. It was a truly empty and incomplete life feeling this way. I did not feel connected to people or pleasures. It was just time marching along.

In my 12-step program, I found out I was not unique, that my food behavior was no different than that of other compulsive overeaters, bulimics, and anorexics. What we shared was compulsive food behavior. I learned that this condition is an illness (though not necessarily viewed as such by the medical community or the world at large). The common misconception is that it is all about will power. That is so not true. People would say just stop, push back from the table, moderation—it does not work when the mind deems otherwise.

The truth is we cannot stop eating altogether. Healthy eating is an issue of choices. And people historically make bad choices. With drugs, alcohol, gambling and sex, the addict can abstain 100 percent if they choose to. The food addict must abstain in moderation. Food must be used to nourish the body. Deciding what foods and how much is appropriate is the challenge. I did not learn to make good food choices as a child. As early as nine, I was told I did not deal with food correctly—I should eat small portions and not want sugary things. Not why, just that I was wrong with my choices. So the more something was denied me, the more I wanted it. And thus the dynamic was set.

Food and I have a love/hate relationship. I loved it and hated it in the same mouthful. But once I started eating, reason left my mind because food always gave me peace. I was fortunate that I rarely suffered from my eating compulsion by being sick or having other kinds of reactions. I hid food everywhere so that I could have what I wanted when I wanted it.

Having the bariatric surgery did change what I had in the home, food-wise. Yes, I bought less food and more appropriate food. The good food was protein and vegetables. But I still bought junk food, items that were small and easy to digest, such as cookies, chips, ice cream, chocolate, and popcorn. The lines got blurred and I made bad choices and the weight returned. At this point, early 2013, I had gained about 60 pounds back. I was having issues with my clothing and I was slowing down. I was so angry with myself: I had taken such an irreversible step and then was sabotaging myself every day!

I was still looking for work and got a call for a job. I went on the interview in June 2013 on a Thursday and was asked to start the next day. It was a contract position to run to the end of the year. Pay was great, I knew someone at the company (the person who recommended me), and I could handle the work. The only possible fly in the ointment was that the company was up for sale. A sale could result in job eliminations, and rumors were that a buyer was in the works and an announcement was eminent.

I was there three weeks when the sale was announced. At the start of my fourth week, the HR manager came up to me and sat me down. He told me that the person I had replaced had appealed to the vice president to get his job back. The vice president had agreed and that meant my contract would be ending. Total SHOCK! I finished my fifth week and was out of work.

And so I ate.

Summer was upon me and I liked having the summer off, but to go through the unemployment process again was depressing. During this time I was still going to therapy and working on issues. Once again, the idea of dealing with my weight and emotional issues was presented and I pretended to be focused.

In November 2013, I got a part-time job doing recruiting for a Detroit-based IT company and I worked partially at home and at the office. I did not like the job but felt I needed to work. Again I avoided taking care of myself. I really felt the "imprint" of what my parents and society expected of me, and that was to work all the time and be a "productive" person. I did not know how to be in tune with myself and to take care of myself consistently. My therapist had been religiously telling me to put myself first, and I fought every thought and action of that for years. Once again, I retreated to a more comfortable space of working constantly in order to avoid dealing with my health.

I was still looking for a full-time job and at the beginning of January 2014; I got an offer, which I accepted. I became a resource manager, meaning I was recruiting staff for our clients. I soon found out that the job wasn't represented well in the interview process and that I had much more work than I had anticipated. I figured that it was still a growth opportunity, and tried to work within the confines of the job so as not to make waves.

Culturally and operationally, I differed with the owner on recruiting methods and hiring approach. The stress grew and I started bringing junk food to eat to soothe my tension during the day. It started small with nuts and Tootsie Rolls. It escalated to chocolate and licorice almost daily. And I was drinking soda pop regularly. Eventually, I had gained so much weight I had to buy new clothes.

My work hours changed, which impacted the drive time coming home. Traffic was much worse later in the day and that created an underlying resentment toward my boss. I don't express anger well or approach the person I have an issue with. I tend to hold things in. So my feelings got twisted and I ate. My brain said I deserved a treat because I was being mistreated. Surgery did not fix this problem. I did not handle this problem with good food choices. I gave in to the feelings.

In June 2014, I expressed concern to a coworker about the fact we had not had any hires with the current clients and the intermediaries we worked with. That night, I got a call saying I was fired. I was stunned. The coworker shared my concerns with the owner, and since I was not perceived as a "team player," I got the axe. So another summer lay off. My friends thought I was doing this deliberately to enjoy the pool. Not so!

But my morale hit an all-time low. I had gained weight back, been through three different jobs in a year, and was still having hourly, daily, and weekly mental struggles with food. This time I really felt that I'd hit bottom. I was so frustrated with my actions and the decisions I had made. I wanted to feel some emotional relief from decision making and daily living and I was not finding it. My level of energy and hope was nonexistent.

[1] The Daring Way, Copyright © 2013 by Brene Brown, Ver. 11.

The Daring Way

In May 2014, I went to a workshop called "The Daring Way" presented by Brené Brown with my therapist, Dr. Sally Palaian, and a group of women. It was two weekend sessions with one follow-up. For once, the session information stayed with me longer than most. The information divided people into groups and talked about "Showing Up," "Being Seen," and "Living Bravely."

The workshop had an exercise on shame. Shame was a feeling I'd had most of my life but had kept in buried deep inside me. Shame held me hostage. We defined our idea of shame in an exercise. My shame revolved around my efforts to handle my weight all these years. Mind you, I said *"handled"* not "managed." I checked out years ago regarding acknowledging and dealing with my weight issues. Something had shifted, and I realized that I didn't want to see myself as a victim anymore, but rather as a participant.

The workshop talked about whether we were moving *"Away, Toward, or Against"* our issues—because that defined the armor we wore to the outside world. (My words, not Brené Brown's.) Brené Brown divided our world into an arena. The world being our arena had seats that represented "people who send or have sent messages about us, as well as the messages themselves."[1] These seats included

1. The Cheap Seats

2. The Box Seats

3. The Critics Section

4. The Support Section

Brené Brown challenged us to explore our arena, not only for who sat there but where we sat ourselves. This workshop really resonated with me, as I, like many baby boomers, had wondered what I would do when I grew up. The thing is, I am grown up! I can't go back and start over at age 21 or 35 or even 50. My life decisions are not going to change, so I can't look back and say: "What if?" I had to move forward and live in the now. I used to live in the future: when I would be normal, I would do so and so. That stopped. I have to participate in my life as best I can at any given moment.

One goal I had was to write a book. I had started books in several different genres over the years but had never finished one. I started writing about my bariatric experience in 2010, thinking it would be a good success story. When I started sliding up the scale in 2011, I put the book down. However, after the Brené Brown workshop concluded, I decided this would be my focus—finishing the book.

I knew that it did not need to be a "success story" but could be my story. When I originally started writing the book, there were no similar books detailing a Bariatric patient's journey. By 2014, there were several such books available on the topic. I hoped that my story would shed light on the pros and cons of the surgery but also the mental food obsession I still have and struggle with daily.

I finished the first draft at the end of January 2015. It was a very proud moment for me. Putting this story in writing—something others might read and talk about—was truly hard. The next step was sharing it with people to get feedback and advice. This was really SCARY for me! Not only was I telling my story, I was actually talking about my real weight, feelings, and experiences. I was taking the mask of self-confidence off and being vulnerable in an area that I did not talk about with anyone.

Turning 60

I turned 60 in August 2014. At that time, my niece, Julia, announced she was getting married the following June. I have one niece and was very proud of her and her many accomplishments. In addition, she was a truly lovely person. I enjoyed watching her grow up and participated in many of her specials moments. Her education, career, and adventures continued to amaze me as well as her future husband, Phil.

I decided to deal with my current health status. I realized that sitting around and thinking about doing something was not going to achieve it. I looked up a fitness-training center I had gone to years ago, Peak Physique. When I went there and talked to the owner, I saw that the overall approach had remained the same and it seemed like a place where I could team up with a trainer and start over. At this time I was still going to therapy biweekly.

I signed up for 10 initial sessions and started two days later. I was scared. I had no idea what I could or could not do physically. I knew that I had gained weight but not how much because I refused to purchase a scale. I weighed in at 344 pounds, and I was actually relieved at that number, as I thought it would be worse. I had kept off 95 pounds of the original 175-pound loss in the last five years. Bariatric surgery is considered successful if you keep off 50% of your weight loss goal. So I would have been considered a success at this point. But I knew I still had a ways to go.

I gradually started working out with a trainer three times a week. Since I was still unemployed, I figured why not? It was hard. It was difficult. But I kept going back. In addition to the physical exercise, the trainer had me write down everything I ate. I was also told to do the following:

1. Limit myself to one piece of fruit per day before noon.

2. Consume any carbs before noon.

3. Get protein before and after a workout.

4. Avoid cheese.

5. Limit bread or eliminate it altogether.

6. Drink lots of water.

7. Avoid soda pop and carbonated drinks.

8. Try to end the day's eating with vegetables or salad.

This was nothing unusual, but it meant that I had to change what I ate and when. I wrote down the food as well as the time because I forget to eat. I rarely sense hunger as a result of the surgery and can often ignore food, but that doesn't work when you're working out hard—you have to feed your body to process what it needs. Plus, forgetting to eat affects my emotional state, and a balanced metabolism helps my overall moods stay in check. I don't stress as much if I eat regularly.

Cheese was the hardest for me to give up. But processed cheese is really unhealthy. I loved sharp cheddar cheese. I bought it on sale and had a least 10 pounds of it in the freezer. Luckily, I found a neighbor who loved it too and could give it away to him. (No way could I throw it away!) I won't say

I am 100 percent off cheese, but I'm pretty darn close. I also have eliminated bread and soda pop from my eating (I say eating rather than diet). The biggest help was writing down the time I ate, which really keeps me focused on eating enough food, especially protein. Not only did I need protein to work out, I needed to keep my bariatric surgery digestive process working well by eating enough protein daily (60–80 grams a day minimally).

I had two trainers in the beginning, Nick, the owner, and then later Lissa. Both were kind, helpful, and encouraging. I was not embarrassed at my skill level and could take in their suggestions without getting resentful. My progress was really showing as the months passed. It was a great experience.

Working out was hard. I came home with pain in body parts I did not know I had. Glutes, triceps, abs—these were new words to me. When soreness or pain showed up, I wanted to know what to do to avoid it, but Lissa told me that soreness meant the body was paying attention to the activity and that was a good thing. Lissa was about 34, a mother of three, and this was her first fitness training job. We bonded over humor and life experiences.

Every sixth session, I got weighed and the weight starting coming off. The more I stayed aware and focused on my food plan, the better it worked. After three months of working out, I had lost 26 pounds. Soon after, I got cocky and lazy, thinking the exercise would carry me if I strayed. And boy did I stray. Ice cream slipped through in the form of Skinny Cow ice cream sandwiches. I did not eat just one; once in a while, I would eat the six pack in one or two days at the most. Bread snuck back in too. There was no surprise that I gained two pounds pretty quickly.

Again, my food-addictive mind played games. I'm losing weight—let's have a treat to celebrate! CRAZY! And I started drinking soda pop again. Self-sabotage rearing its head and the food addiction was doing push-ups in the parking lot. Whenever I got cocky about my progress, I would think of a way to revert back to old eating habits.

The other issue was boredom. I still was not working and felt restless about not having more to do. I was fortunate that I was collecting unemployment. I felt that I should be doing more. My therapist reminded me that this was a good time to take care of me so I would be better equipped down the road. She said: "Why not take advantage of the time and work your program?" That did not eliminate the restlessness. I was still attending 12-step program meetings all the while and that helped distract and focus me.

Christmas 2014

Christmas was approaching and I was really worried about handling holiday eating. I was asked to make some family-favorite cookies to bring to dinner and I agreed, which was maybe not the smartest move. But I decided I could handle it. I made two recipes: walnut refrigerator cookies and petticoat tails cookies. I must have been sorely out of practice baking because the end result was horrible. I had to throw them out. I think I had forgotten how to bake. I thought God was having fun with me and found it hilarious. Glad that someone was looking out for me when I was not.

I asked a neighbor to help me try again and between us we made petticoat tails and shortbread and Russian tea cake cookies. I also made chocolate chip cookies—just the single-serving recipe—and immediately put them in tins in the garage to keep cold. I had no real desire for any of them. So I survived the holiday pretty well and felt like I was back on track.

Another change I made was to ask John and his wife, Kate, who were staying with me over the holidays, what they wanted to eat. I could get their items and not have extra "just in case" things like snacks. This method worked really well, and I knew if they wanted something specific, they could go get it themselves. Overall, it was a good exercise in planning for me. Plus I was practicing the "new me" who took care of her needs—and herself!

One issue I had to deal with was people giving me food as gifts over the holidays. These were people that knew I struggled with weight and food, yet they still gave me treats and sugary items. Most of them went down the garbage disposal, and some were handed off to others. I appreciated the gesture, but realized how we have forgotten to socialize when food isn't the main focus.

January 2015 had been a bit of a rough ride, as I'd been having trouble staying on my food plan. I realized that I had also stopped writing my food down and having accountability with my trainer. Out of sight, out of mind, I thought to myself. I had to renew my efforts to get moving in the right direction. My goal is to continue to show up!

Part of that effort was joining another fitness center that offered a great pool. I LOVE to swim. I like doing water aerobics and know that I can do some things in the water easier than on land. I went to check out the pool at the Sola Fitness Center (part of Beaumont hospital system) and joined at the end of December. I now swim about three to four times a week in addition to my fitness workouts. The workouts have greatly strengthened me overall. When I started, using a 5-pound weight was hard; now I'm working out with 15 pounds weights. My balance is greatly improved, and I have more core body strength. Peak Physique continues to challenge and encourage me in this effort and I am grateful.

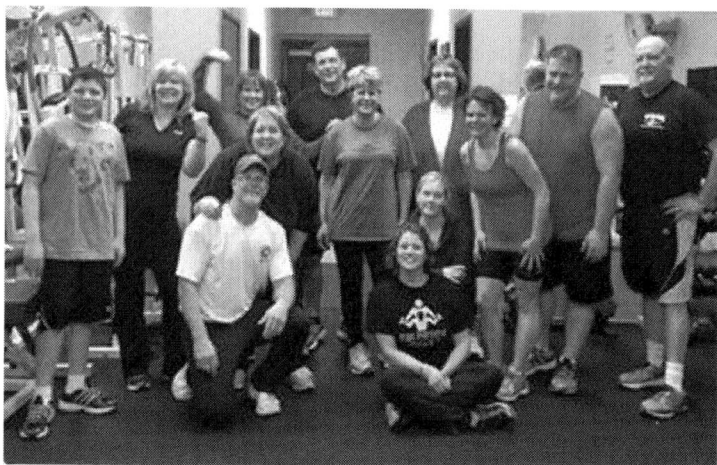

You must think that by now I have my act together and everything is going great. I wish it were that simple. I still have everyday emotional issues, which trigger my food obsession. Just this last week I knew I was off-center, uneasy and unhappy. I couldn't really figure out the issue, but knew I could solve it if I got a Saunders birthday cake (vanilla cake, butter cream frosting and nuts on the side). I told myself that it would make the feelings go away and I would be fine. I have thought about that cake for over a week and still want it even though I now know what triggered these thoughts. How silly is it to obsess over a cake for more than a week? And the problem is, I am still scared I might go get it and try to eat the whole thing in one sitting.

That is why gastric bypass surgery is just one of the many tools in the box I can use to control food issues. It is not the "cure" or the "cop" to manage my food. There is no cure. There is no 24 hour bodyguard in the kitchen.

When I celebrated a successful sales deal, I would binge on a pizza or a lot of chocolate. If I survived an uncomfortable event socially, I would eat something sugary like cookies or brownies. A local bakery was a favorite for loading up with treats after a particularly bad day. I always said I was buying for the office but I am sure they did not care one way or another.

For 2016, my small and attainable goals were:

1. Continue to lose weight and get healthy,

2. Have surgery to remove excessive stomach skin,

3. Enjoy life to the fullest (do the things I want to without delay: travel, explore new hobbies and activities, eliminate fear if the unknown, etc.)

So far, #3 is winning,

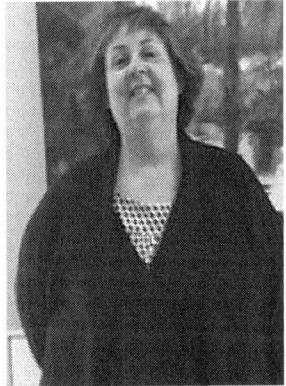

December 2014

Random Thoughts

Food triggers. One food that absolutely sends me into frenzy is commercially manufactured, processed Rice Krispy Treats. I can eat the homemade ones without issue, but put a processed, store-bought version of this item in my mouth and I become a raving lunatic. I cannot eat just one. It triggers a reaction in me that I have never experienced with any other food. First I bought one or two. Then it was six. Then it was the family size of 12–18. I would take these treats to work. If I had one, I would scarf the rest down until they were gone. I could not pace myself. I would eat all of them within an hour easily. And I could still eat more if available. I had to force myself not to buy them. EVER!

As I have progressed through the years post-surgery, I have found that I have had surgical success. The surgeon is happy with my progress; my lab tests are within normal ranges; I have had little difficulty with digestion and food portions—all good. My "tool" worked. That success is just one component of the bigger picture. I can truly say I have had surgical success! But to make weight loss work and stay in place requires a lot more pieces. For me, those pieces are exercise, lifestyle changes, record keeping and problem solving.

Car seat belts. For the first time since I started driving, I can easily put on a seat belt and not just in my car but in any car. You have no idea how that makes me feel! Elation! Relief! I don't have to fumble with the seat belt and no longer have to pretend to be wearing one to avoid a ticket or say I will ride in the back to avoid the requirement of wearing a seat belt in Michigan. And yes, I tried the belt extender but that really did not work, as it didn't feel secure. I no longer have to listen to my mother nag me about wearing a seat belt.

Now I also know that the air bag will deploy properly, since I can tilt the steering wheel back to a standard setting. The actual seat no longer has to be at its maximum extension both in distance and height. This means that I will also have many more car model selections to choose from in the future—woo woo!

Movie seats. Now I can sit comfortably at movies. In the past, if the movie seat had a rigid cup holder armrest, I often would come away with bruises on either side of my stomach from trying to squash myself into the seat. The seat would tilt back so far that it was awkward to sit in and I would place my purse and/or jacket behind my back just to sit upright.

Chairs with arms. I don't have to scan a room or restaurant to see if they have a chair without arms or ask for a table rather than a booth so I won't be embarrassed trying to slide in. I can fit in any booth at this point. I still catch myself asking for a table when going to a restaurant. Each time I slide into a booth, I smile to myself and feel so good.

When I was at the rehab facility in Arizona and went to my first group session, the therapist pointed to a chair without arms as the one for me to sit in. I got so mad about the fact she identified me in front of everyone as needing a chair without arms. I called her on it after the session, stating she was treating me like a child who could not take care of herself when in reality she was trying to be considerate.

This was one example of how I was always on the offensive about anything weight related. My challenge to her help send me to the head therapist, who thought I had issues with authority and wanted to switch me to a different group. I, with my usual "don't give a damn" attitude, pointed out that I did not need someone to remind me I was fat. Definite attitude—if you please! My time there was minimally successful. I went through the motions; I tried to figure out what they (the staff) wanted and go along. But I was still in my protective shell and thinking I could figure things out on my own.

There were some positive aspects of this recovery attempt. I allowed myself to try a new approach to my weight issues. I learned I was not alone. I learned that some of the medical profession believed food addiction was a real disease. I learned that there were other ways of dealing with the root causes of how and why I ate.

Now, I am not saying it all penetrated my pea brain. It just opened up another door and allowed me to think about alternatives for my future, and that helped me with dialogue with my therapist and a few trusted friends. Plus, it was the first time I let my family know how unhappy I was and that I did want to change. Again, I still wanted to be anonymous and paid for this treatment out of my own pocket. I did not tell anyone at work what I was doing except my boss; I just left to go to Arizona.

Dining out. I have found that I can be very specific about my food requirements when ordering. As an obese person, I was painfully aware of the feeling of being watched as I ate and feeling judged, whether it was true or not. Was I eating too much? Was I eating the wrong foods? Could I order dessert? Would the rest of the people order as well so I would not stand out? All these thoughts are what drove me to the drive-through (get the pun?) and other less public dining. If you really take the time to look around in a restaurant, no one pays attention to you and if they do it is brief and forgettable. After you leave, even the wait staff forgets you unless you stiff them on the tip. Too many diners go through the restaurant doors to be remembered by any of the wait staff, unless you are a regular.

Restaurants are providing healthier choices and are aware of health issues like allergies, diabetes, etc., and are more accommodating. Some places will allow you to sample something before ordering. I still bring home leftovers. I often eat the equivalent of an appetizer portion or smaller. Plus, I received a laminated card from Henry Ford Hospital indicating I had had gastric bypass surgery that asks restaurants to serve me a child-sized portion, just in case there was something on the children's menu that appealed to me.

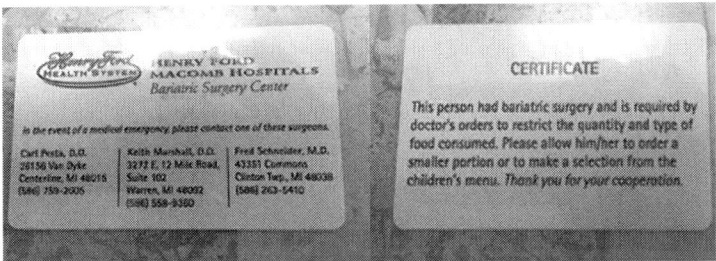

Unfortunately, many restaurants do not honor the card. Many think you just want to buy a kids' meal or do not understand the dietary restrictions.

Tying shoes. As a heavy person, I used to tie my tennis shoes on the inner side because I could only reach it by angling my foot up. I could not bend over my belly and tie the shoe dead center. I notice I don't do this anymore.

Traveling. I flew to England in October 2010, and when I compare it to my previous trip in 2007, it was like day and night. I could walk. I could walk a lot. I was not tired all the time. I was willing to venture out and about and not be embarrassed. I actually bought some clothes in Cambridge.

Weigh yourself. It is recommended that you should weigh yourself only once a week and when looking at your results, compare them over a four-week period. I know when I was in rapid weight loss during those first few months, I hit a week where I plateaued, and I was shocked and mad. But the Henry Ford nurse coordinator asked me to look back at my weight loss for the last four weeks, and I realized that I had lost 18 pounds. She gently reminded me that I would eventually slow down and experience plateaus and, when I hit those plateaus, to review what actions were occurring and adjust accordantly.

Hunger. Define hunger: head, stomach, or heart hunger. There is not just one kind of hunger. Normal people have stomach hunger. Dysfunctional people have all kinds of hunger. In order to soothe my different hungers, I ate, because that was what I knew. I learned to squash my feelings and eat rather than dealing with the issue in front of me. I used to drink soda all day rather than eat. When I stopped doing that, it was still hard to know whether I felt physical hunger or emotional hunger. With the surgery, I don't feel stomach hunger at all, and I have to remind myself to eat. Emotions still trigger the thought to eat, but not stomach hunger.

Success. Fear of success. Losing the weight may be the primary object but for a long time, lack of weight loss kept me safe. I didn't not have to reach too high, be more outgoing, and try harder. I had a lot of dreams as a young adult. I wanted to be a photojournalist or join the navy, neither of which I did. I wrote a play when I was eleven and wanted to write more. I wanted to write a TV sitcom (still do). I wanted to write a book (I did). There are many things I set aside because I was fat. I did not feel safe enough to try my dreams. The weight defined me.

I had success in other areas. Sales, work, friends, but not always the things that nurture your soul. I have traveled extensively, domestically and internationally. I have been white-water rafting, ridden in a hot air balloon, gone on cruises, lived in Hawaii for almost a year—things most people don't get to try. I thought that was enough. As the weight came off, I became aware of so many more things I want to experience in life—more travel, maybe do a marathon of some kind, take a yoga class comfortably, etc.

While the surgery helped me create new boundaries, it also opened my mind and attitude to "What's next?" I feel less limited or scared to try new things—not just physical activities but creative ones like writing this book, doing video work, maybe painting again.

Reflections

As I pass the seven-year mark of my surgery, I feel fortunate that it has worked well for me. I have learned that it is not a guarantee to weight loss, that my food choices still impact my success or failure rate, that people still judge you by appearance, and all of that is less important than being happy and healthy.

I have noticed that my hair has improved—both the texture and body have returned to 80 percent of the way they were. It had been very dry and thin looking for most of the first two years after the surgery. Another improvement is that I am no longer cold all the time. Out of habit, I was wearing a sweater every day, and one day I realized I did not need it. So my internal thermometer is getting back to normal.

I have new bulges, though. Decorating or covering these defined bulges is harder than draping my bulk before. I thought I could hide the entire package. Silly me. Oversized shirts did not really hide the bulk—I just thought it did. My legs and arms are a normal size, but now my middle is this lumpy mess. I have tried a Spanx-type clone garment, which is really uncomfortable and hard to get on or off. I sure don't want to resort to the old days of a girdle, but I need to find a solution. Oh well. If that is the worst I have to deal with, I will survive.

Changing my attitude has been an evolution that took many years, and therapy has played a huge role in it. The consistency of my therapist's support and her belief in me made the steps I took less scary and more doable than they would have been without her help. I do not honestly think I would have taken the steps to heal myself on many levels without Dr. Sally Palaian. Sally is a kind, compassionate person who has stuck with me through all the denial, fear, frustration, and acceptance. She offered me many alternatives to work through my issues, helped me take baby steps when needed and bigger ones when I was ready. Dr. Palaian is someone I trust completely but I don't always agree with, and that is okay.

I appreciate that as Dr. Palaian incorporates new techniques in her practice she makes them available to me. I have tried several things like breathwork, eye movement desensitization and reprocessing, the Brené Brown workshop, and others in my journey. I took away something from each technique that pushed me along my path.

Some of the things I learned were that what matters to oneself is important, and so is taking the time to listen to one's body and desires. If I continue to fill that space with busywork or frantic chaos, I do myself a disservice and abandon the care of keeping me well. The only one who can truly know what I need is myself, and if I can let others into my life, I can reach out for help without shame or guilt and get what I need.

For a very long time, I refused to express my feelings other than anger because I thought I needed to be strong. As long as I chugged away and worked and worked and achieved, then I was a success. I made lots of money, traveled the world, tried many exciting things, but was unhappy and alone. The emotional bond or connection I desired wasn't there. I did not know how to make one, so I turned to food. Ah, food! Cheap, fast, abundant, and very accessible. If you didn't see me eat it, then I didn't. That's how a food addict's mind works.

Food Addict. Yes, I said it. Food Addict! God, I hate those words. I feel such a failure when I hear them. I did not want this tag, this label anywhere near me. I thought it made me ugly, ashamed, guilty, dirty, and so much more. And it is not the word "food" but rather the word "addict" that I cringe at. "Addict" meant such horrible things in my mind—homeless, dirty, disgusting, weak—all sorts of things that I avoided and feared. I really had little reference or exposure to any kind of addict while growing up.

But what I really feared was the emotions that the addiction hid. In my little pot of crazy was shame, fear, guilt, longing, loneliness, and more. Somewhere as a child, I learned (i.e., felt) that I was not whole, that somehow I was lacking, and from that point on, worked at trying to fix me to be acceptable to the adults around me. I took on a personality that put on a brave front while I felt like I was dying inside. I was a clown, a good student, a Camp Fire Girl, a Girl Scout, a tomboy—so many roles that I forgot the little one inside and tucked her away into what I believed safety was. When asked to describe the little one, I always said she is in my bedroom closet, hiding in the dark, in the corner, trying to be smaller or invisible.

For years, I tried to be smaller. I felt I took up more space than I should and felt embarrassed when noticed. Sitting on a bus or plane, I always notice the looks given to me because I took up more space than a normal-sized person. No one wanted to share a partial seat with me. To get close to others, I would take on roles, chores, or responsibilities that were unnecessary, and I took on adult roles way too soon, all the while thinking that if I lightened others' burdens, it would give them time to be with me. Unfortunately, a child's reality and thought process is just that—a child's. And there was no way to cope with adult issues and interactions.

I never stopped trying. Entering my 20s and 30s, I thought I was the family mediator and I tried to keep everyone happy, encouraged outings, and gave lots of gifts to show how much I cared. I was definitely overly generous with my time and money. I was convinced that showering people with gifts and outings would draw them to me. I placed a much higher value on these things than others did and was always disappointed afterwards when the relationship balance stayed the same. Relationships were a game for me. I mentally kept score and tried to stay one step or point ahead at all times. It was EXHAUSTING.

The harder I tried, the worse outcomes I attained. I would get so angry that people did not fall over me all the time. Through therapy and much conversation, I saw that my reality of relationships was very childish. I thought people valued the same things I did and would get frustrated when they did not gush over what I had done or react the way I wanted them to. I had a habit of being self-contained and rigid, projecting an aura that sometimes people were not drawn to, one that they tiptoed around. Somehow I wanted to be the bright light that people were drawn to like a moth to a flame. When that did not happen, I got bitter. And that bitterness grew. And the volume of food eaten grew, to the point that I made myself sick.

I ate when I felt out of control over my feelings, a work situation, a person, a social event, whatever . . . Once I opened a package, I felt compelled to finish the entire thing, even if it wasn't my favorite or even didn't taste that good. I had to get my "value," and that is when I knew my food obsession crossed over into the money realm.

If I was going to binge, I damn well was going to get value and use a coupon or get two-for-one items. I looked for marked-down items, day-old goods, or cheap versions of name brands. My insane rationalization made me think that because I got a "deal" on an item, it wasn't so bad if I ate all of it. Absurd! But an addict's mind is very creative and will do anything to get its drug, so you become this force of nature that is hard to slow, much less stop.

Even now after the surgery, I still have the same mentality. If I cheat, I still like the "twos" (two bags of cookies, candies, chips) and I still use coupons, still look at the marked-down goods. Surgery does not cure the mind; it just creates different consequences. I try to avoid stores like Big Lots, Target, Costco, and Sam's Club so I am not tempted to buy big bags of anything sweet or chocolaty. Little thoughts of "will I get enough food" when I am at social functions or family events still creep into my head. I still take leftovers home, and that can amount to two or three more meals.

Recently, I went to Ridley's, which is a bakery and sandwich shop. I had a coupon from the Entertainment Book, and I ordered a chicken salad and tuna salad sandwich without the bread. The sandwiches came with coleslaw and a tiny brownie. But it was two for one . Again, the insane mentality kicked in. I wanted a cookie because I saved money on the sandwiches. I actually mulled over my choices until I realized what I was doing and got the heck out of there!

I want to live to a fairly old age. For a long time I could not see a future and especially my future because I was just existing and going through the motions of life—sleep, eat, work, sleep, eat, work, rest—which is not a real life by any means, and to think of doing that for the next 30–40 years—no way.

I realize I will have stress. I realize that there will be situations I cannot handle by myself. I realize that I have emotions but I also have control as to how I react to those emotions.

The Economic Impact of Obesity

The economic impact of being overweight is overwhelming when you break it down. The obvious costs are food, clothes, and health care. But the additional financial concerns impact a person's furniture, cars, housing, jobs, travel, social interactions, and much more. After surgery, I immediately noticed that my food costs went down, and I had less doctor visits. I have more options with clothing and am able to take advantage of items at greatly reduced prices in a much broader range of stores. I don't have to buy only through catalogs or online. I love that! My health and life insurance rates dropped. (I can get life insurance now.) I can purchase standard furniture—not reinforced items. I can buy a scale because the range of it works for me. It is less likely that I will develop diabetes, high blood pressure, or heart disease (I said LESS likely). I have already seen an improvement in my asthma and arthritis.

I don't have to buy "specialty" items, which typically can cost 25–50 percent more. I don't worry when I visit friends that I might not find a chair I can sit in comfortably without embarrassment. I used to look for chairs without arms at friends', restaurants, theatres, etc. An old embarrassing moment was when I was a teen and was at an aunt's home and broke the wooden toilet seat in one of the bathrooms. I was so mortified. I tried to act as if nothing happened and did not inform anyone that the seat was broken. I never admitted it to anyone before today.

Travel is cheaper and more convenient. At a lower weight, I feel more comfortable traveling and utilizing specialty sites or theme parks because I can participate. I can manage the walking and the bumping and jostling of the crowds with greater ease and patience.

Interviewing for jobs is easier, and this slimmer body goes over a lot better than the old one that would huff and puff walking down a hallway. My body image is more professional and capable. It is all about perception. But the funny thing is that for the job I just landed at Kelly Services, all the interviewing was conducted over the telephone (not even Skype) and there was not one session in person.

I can't wait to replace my driver's license this year and get a new picture, as both my driver's license and passport have old pictures that show me as much heavier. I don't want to be accused of having a fake ID when it is checked!

Cosmetic Surgery

I treated myself to cosmetic surgery to remove my bat wings, or excess skin on my arms. I had not worn sleeveless tops in a very long time and wanted to feel good about my weight loss progress. I consulted a plastic surgeon, Dr. Vik Reddy, in February 2015 in order to plan this event. I wanted to have the surgery and be healed prior to my niece's wedding.

After the initial consultation, surgery was booked for April 2015, and healing time was approximately three to four weeks. I asked my oldest brother, Paul, to come and help me out during the recovery time. At the time of surgery, I had been working out for about six months and was feeling great.

Outpatient surgery took place on April 27. I was out like a light and woke up in recovery. I came home and after two days stopped the pain medication. My follow-up visit on April 29 was great. Another visit on May 1 let me drive since I was off pain medication. On May 8 I was allowed to resume swimming and I was working out again the following week. It went incredibly smoothly.

**BEFORE -
4/27/2015**

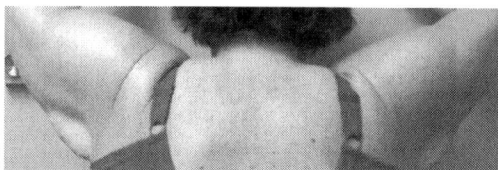

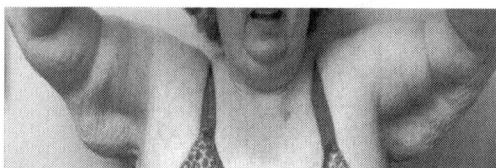

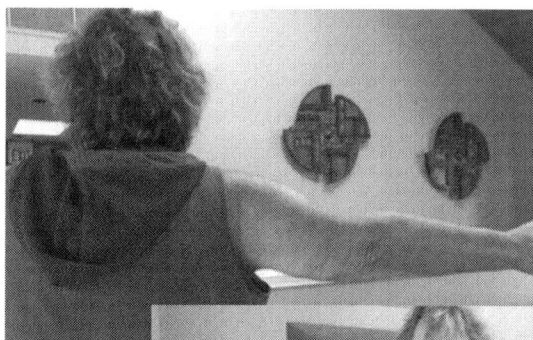

**AFTER
7/2015**

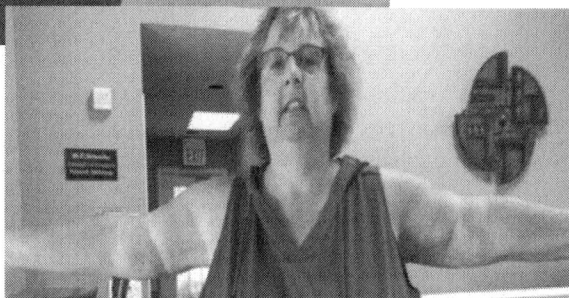

I wore two different sleeveless dresses for the family wedding and was thrilled to pieces. I thoroughly enjoyed the summer wearing new tops and showing off my arms.

Summary—Maybe

Here I am still trying to learn to face my pain and emptiness. The process is rough, and sometimes overwhelming. What I've noticed is that I no longer go immediately to food for comfort. I turned to food almost unconsciously before surgery. I would only realize what I had done after about half a bag of chocolate or box of Cheez-Its. It got to a point that any emotion caused me to feel overwhelming "hunger." I didn't even let my brain decide what kind of feelings I had; all I knew was that I wanted to feel nothing, and food gave me this escape, so I emotionally ate and numbed out.

As I learn new ways of coping, I am forced to face my feelings. I've had to actually talk about issues, to let myself get angry. What I am most surprised about is that my feelings haven't overwhelmed me; I didn't die and I didn't disappear. Shame! I needed to resolve my existing internalized shame. I still held on to shame over many big and small items. Sometimes it is about not being able to cope, the overwhelming feelings I get and how I handle them or just not feeling "good enough." Thank goodness for therapy, my 12-step program and perseverance. I felt ashamed that I could not control my eating. I was successful at controlling so many other things, why did this elude me. I knew it was self-destructive, but food was the only thing that stopped my emotional pain. I wasn't even sure what the pain was from anymore. All I knew was that it was a kind of emptiness, a feeling of being abandoned and alone. I use food to solve pain.

I have found that my journey to health and wellness is truly a daily struggle. I must exercise; watch my diet, vitamin, and fluid intake; and practice gratitude, acceptance, forgiveness, love, and hope. My life and health depends on all of these elements.

My addiction still exists and will never go away. I must continue to understand myself and my emotional needs so I do not gain my weight back, or at least sabotage a further weight loss. I believed that something emotional within me triggers my need to eat and I can destroy myself. The key to dealing with my food addiction is avoidance of trigger foods. Food addiction can eventually override my gastric bypass surgery, if I let it.

I thought this was where I would end my book. While I was working on the finishing touches on this book, my niece, Julia, got married, I reunited with a man from my past and a relationship evolved into an engagement, I experienced a bizarre employer and guilt, and then got a great job, then lost it. Life continues. So does this story.

Julia's Wedding and After

I felt so great at the wedding. My clothes fit well, and I was very mobile and able to keep up with all the activities. But after five days in Chicago and all of the parties, I was ready to come home. There was a bit of a letdown, as the event I had worked so hard to get ready for (lose weight, have surgery, find clothes, etc.) was over. I had to set some new goals.

Distraction occurred and my goals were put on the shelf. I started a new job as a full-time recruiter just before the wedding and when I got back, I had high hopes with my new employer. I quickly learned I was entering the danger zone. I thought being on the ground floor of a company restarting and repositioning itself would be to my advantage. I would have a chance to create my role and be part of the next iteration of the business. It was a small business and family owned. As I tried to do my job, I was continually challenged by small unwritten and unspoken rules. (I could not use out-of-state candidates, American or green card holders only, the family wanted to interview my candidates prior to presenting to client, etc.) I felt blindsided and restricted in my efforts. I started eating in between my planned meals. Little things at first, like miniature Tootsie Rolls. I would bring in a large bag of them, planning to ration the candy over a long period of time. They barely lasted three to four days. Then it was popcorn, and then anything I thought would calm me. I started gaining weight and I was struggling again.

At the same time love entered my life in late July 2015. A lovely man began to pursue me. I was quite surprised. We had met eight years before, and at that time he was married. A mutual business contact of ours called me and asked if they could give him my telephone number, as he had asked to contact me. I didn't think much about the request at the time and said yes. This was on a Thursday, and he, Pat, called me on Sunday night. He was now divorced and said he had thought of me often over the years. We made plans to meet for lunch the following Saturday. I have to admit that I didn't remember what he looked like. I called our mutual contact. She described Pat to me, but I still could not quite picture his face in my mind.

We met for lunch. I recognized him, and he was very cute! He seemed shy and quiet—not something I am used to in my friends. Lunch went well and we made plans to talk later in the week. I figured I had nothing to lose and would gain a friend. (When I first met Pat eight years ago, I was at least 100 pounds heavier than I was at this meeting.) My weight was not an issue to him.

We started seeing each other every week, usually at a park in the evening to enjoy the sunshine. I didn't feel like I had to have a meal to have a date and this technique worked. Pat is a massage therapist and had recently returned to the area. He was starting his business up again and did not have money to spend on outings anyway. Things progressed, and we began dating regularly. He would come visit me at work sometimes, and I now had a witness to my work insanity (massive amount of furniture, files, knickknacks, paper, general clutter, etc.).

Summer merged into fall, work and Pat kept me busy. But my eating suffered. I was stressed in new ways and was returning to old habits. I started drinking soda again—which is by far the WORST thing I did. My emotional stability was looking and feeling like a roller coaster. I was tiptoeing in a job that was a minefield and I had a man who seemed intent on being my boyfriend. I think I could have handled one or the other well, but not both.

By October, Pat was a constant in my life and meals were becoming a challenge. When we got together on Friday evenings, I initially cooked a meal and we spent the evening together. But now Pat wanted to go out or order pizza on Fridays. I tried to make that work for me. It did not. Sometimes I could not find a safe or comfortable food to consume. Other times we would order something and split it, and I would be resentful because I could not eat an equal portion and felt cheated (both cost- and food-wise). My food plan got muddled. I brought food items for Pat and then they became items for me too. The lines got blurred.

I started baking again so that I could impress Pat and would send food home with him and have some for myself. I cooked foods that I would normally do for family events under the premise of sharing my cooking talents with him. I baked more items that holiday season than I had in years. Volume and frequency became an issue (my just-in-case food scenarios).

In November, work took a turn for the worse and I resigned. I was upset with myself, frustrated at the overall situation and just plain mad at the world. At the same time, I had a major hiccup with Pat. So I turned to food. You would think with my 12-step program, therapy, and previous success, relapses would be less frequent. Trust me, there is one around every corner. Once I stopped working, I upped my workouts to four or five a week. I had maintained my exercise routine while I worked: cross-fit two times a week and swimming twice a week. I tried to add additional sessions to combat the weight I had put on, and it worked for a while.

During this time, I also signed up for a class to become certified as a "soul coach," a professional life coach, beginning the intro course in October 2015. I enjoyed it and started my own coaching practice in November. My business is named willing2becoached. As part of the class, we had to do pro bono work with clients, a minimum of five hours. I also had some paying clients. I loved this work.

I enrolled in the advance soul coach class that started in January 2016. I received certification in March 2016. This class and coaching kept me busy though the next few months. As part of my effort to expand my business, I took classes at the local public access TV station for our city and county. First was video camera operation, then studio equipment, and finally editing. Initially, I filmed three episodes of myself coaching a guest named Sue. I used those episodes as my practice. One of my other coaches, Scott, asked if I would videotape him practicing a speech for Toastmasters. From that evolved four more shows, coaching vignettes by Scott F.

Pat got a little jealous about the time I was spending with other coaches and filming. He asked me to help him in a martial arts–themed shoot. That was my next project. From this work, more has come in and it is an ongoing effort, which I really enjoy. The shows are broadcasted on public access TV on Channel 18 in my city. The hosts get a copy to use as their own (on YouTube, Facebook or their own website).

My relationship was deepening, and Pat and I were moving forward. I had many reservations and fears. One was that Pat is fourteen years younger than I am. He is okay with the age difference, but it took me a little longer to be comfortable. Age was not the only twist, as a man had not called me pretty or beautiful in many years. And while my weight was down, I did not feel pretty. I felt closer to normal, but not pretty.

I've always had great self-esteem; school, work, and social life were not challenges. Relationships were. I had closed myself off to the possibilities of a relationship long ago and I had been alone for the last several years with no man on the horizon. Now Pat had showed up. He was totally accepting and appreciative of me just how I was, not asking me to change physically. But I had to work hard to believe this. It was difficult for me to see what he saw and accept it. He saw a sexy, pretty, confident woman. I could grasp the "confident" part. (I still am working the acceptance part.)

Additionally, there was some adjustment. I had to learn to consider another person's feelings. I was so accustomed to doing what I wanted when I wanted that I came across as arrogant at times. I was not used to sharing my world with another. Sometimes frustration or impatience crept in and those were food triggers in the past. I had a slippery slope to traverse. I was learning to act as part of a couple rather than a lone ranger. Sometimes I got confused in the couple role.

Pat was a "late" person—he stayed up late and rose later in the morning than I did. I am an early riser, usually awake and moving by 6:00 a.m. Being tired from the different schedules and naturally busy contributed to my lapse in food planning. My normal meal planning on Sunday got sloppy and incomplete. I was eating out more, making not-so-safe choices, and not thinking about my overall health. This continued into the spring, and I finally felt the result when I pulled out summer clothes and could not fit into my shorts.

I was pretty devastated. The remainder of my weight is in my stomach area, and I have the sagging apron of fat left there. Weight I gained had returned to this area, making my clothes too small. At first, I was pissed at myself, knowing perfectly well why this happened. Lack of attention to my food plan and bad decisions adds up.

Knowing that I had to change, I sat Pat down and told him that I had to make changes. I could no longer go out to eat so much. I had to cook more. I had to eliminate soda altogether to be sane. He said he would work with that. Pat, too, had felt the effects of our eating, gaining more than 25 pounds. He did go to one 12- step program meeting with me, but didn't see himself as a compulsive overeater.

Pat gave me a bicycle to use, and when I tried to ride it, I had a hard time with the pedals. They were in the standard position but that was too close to the frame for me. Because my weight is in my stomach and thighs, I could not keep my feet inward and on the pedals. I needed to have them extended so I could plant my feet more firmly. I was embarrassed but could admit what I needed. Pat was disappointed but did not have a solution. This is a difficulty facing overweight people in day-to-day living. Even when we can identify the issue, there is not always a remedy.

Pat is supportive and liked to walk and work out, but we were not doing that together. He does martial arts, yoga, and the like. I am not much for walking but do the treadmill and workout regularly at a fitness center. We have talked about working out together but our schedules are so different, we still have not done it together. Swimming is my preferred sport. My knees and ankles have supported me for years but tend to need gentle treatment now.

Our relationship continues to evolve. We got engaged in August 2016. I am not sure I want to have a real marriage in the sense of a legal arrangement. I am a little set in my ways and like the flexibility of being single. Pat was married and prefers that commitment. Time will tell whether we go to the next level.

The idea of a celebration would be great! I would get to dress up and party with family and friends, so we have discussed a Buddhist commitment ceremony. Pat is in charge of figuring that out. For now, we are spending more time together, I am practicing honesty in my feelings and moods, and we talk about issues right away so that no one stays hurt or angry. These are all actions that have been reinforced by being in a 12-Step Program.

Cuba

In mid-spring 2016, I also took off to Cuba with friends from Canada. We had talked about going in January 2016, but that trip was cancelled due to a family death of one of the group. We regrouped and went in March 2016. Instead of 12, there was just 4 of us. From Windsor, Ontario, direct to Varadero, Cuba, was a three-hour flight, on which free food and drinks were served and a movie was shown (both ways). Upon arrival, we bused to our all-adult, all- inclusive resort and settled in for a week.

In a weird way, food was easier to handle in Cuba. The resort did not provide room service, and meals were provided three times a day in the dining room and served buffet style. There was a wide assortment of choices, plenty to choose from in order to make safe selections. So I was limited in the times I could eat, and as a result, I did make better food choices and ate consistently for most of the week. There was a store on the premises, which had some snacks, but not a wide variety.

On top of this, taking two different day trips did not lend itself to eating badly. Lunch was provided as part of the tour but was generally chicken, vegetable, and some desert. Basic choices. The stores in Cuba did not have a wide variety of things and stocked very few American brands. A can of Coke was three dollars. I could focus on relaxing and not the food. I still had crazy food thoughts, just no way to act on them. I spent very little money on souvenirs except for coffee and honey, which I gave as gifts to friends and family.

While in Cuba, I took a fall, hitting my shoulder, knee, and head. The left knee swelled like a baseball but quick icing and drugs controlled the pain and damage. The shoulder, however, did not flare up until I got home and that lingered for three weeks. I could barely raise my arm. Pain equals food. Another setback. I wish I had remembered to work my 12-step program. But I have to say that by working out, I bounced back more quickly than I had after past falls.

When I returned home, I attempted to resume my food plan. I had left town after a small fight with Pat and wasn't looking forward to working through my problems. It was still gloomy in Michigan and those seemed like good excuses to not eat wisely. Plus my regular trainer, Debbie A., was out of town (I was out of sorts), I was sore from my fall, and I needed to take time off, all elements that I let undermine my program.

A food addict (me) will always rationalize the bad decisions. I began to be sloppy with my food plan and veer off into bad choices and not eat enough protein.

Summer 2016

Summer is fast approaching and it will be swimming weather. I don't want people to see that I have regained some weight but a bathing suit hides very little. I won't give up my swimming, and never have at any weight. I finally broke down and purchased some shorts in a larger size. They are a reminder of where I currently am at.

I know that I must live in the present and be aware if I am to change and improve. Some days are better than others. Life happens, and how I handle it is still up to me. Looking back, I am happy I made the decision to have the surgery. It saved my life.

So my status right now is that I have kept off 120 pounds, still working out trying to lose more weight. I am dealing with food on a daily basis but have a good support system in place (therapy, 12-step, finance, etc.). I am in a good place—great man, great job, doing video and coaching work, enjoying my home and friends. Life is good and my reality is pretty good too. My wish is to lose 20 or more pounds and have the stomach surgery to remove the sagging skin.

Surgical Success

What is success? Surgical success is the patient did not die or have complications. If that is the definition, then I am a success story. But that is a bit simplistic. The success is in how the surgical creation of the "tool" works for me. As long as I follow the guidelines, this "tool" should work well and provide the desired effect (i.e., weight loss).

This surgery impacts hormones like ghrelin, which stimulates one's appetite and signals the brain that we should eat and satisfy hunger. In my case, I think I grew that hormone to massive proportions and it ruled my life. Some medical researchers say that process can be crippled by eating junk food or by stress. Junk food's lethal combination of fat, sugar, and salt stimulates dopamine, which then triggers the brain to seek food.

The end ... for now!

I hope that this story offers you insight and hope as you follow your journey.

I would love to hear your story and possibly share it with others in another book. If interested, please email your story to me at:

willing2becoached@gmail.com

– Nicki Travis

Made in the USA
San Bernardino, CA
15 January 2017